Weight Wa

101 Quick and Easy Recipes for Rapid Weight Loss

Madison Miller

ISBN: 978-1535539906

Printed in the United States

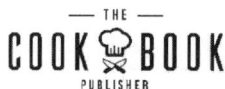

Avant-Propos

What is the most difficult part of following a dietary plan? For most people, it's simply having the time and energy to follow through with healthy eating for every meal and snack, every single day. Even with plans like Weight Watchers®®, which make healthy choices and weight loss incredibly easy, our busy daily lives still make it a struggle. This book has been created to address this very problem with a bounty of delicious solutions. Here you will find recipes that can be created in thirty minutes or less, using five ingredients or fewer. It really doesn't get much simpler than this! Each recipe comes with nutritional information and the Weight Watchers® SmartPoint™ value to help you make eating choices that are best for you. From this point on, fitting nutritious, homemade meals into your schedule does not need to be a problem. Now you can focus on flavor and satisfaction with this delicious collection of easy and simple recipes.

Contents

Introduction

What, in your mind, does it mean to be healthy? Is it about how you feel, how you look, what your outlook on life is? For most of us, healthy is a combination of what goes on inside our bodies and how we present ourselves to the world with our outer appearance. It really doesn't matter if you are someone who has made healthy choices a priority your whole life, or if you are someone who has struggled and is ready for a new start, each of us can say that we are bombarded with different dietary plans and trends. Some "diets" are complicated, others claim to be based on our primitive means of survival, and a new trend is health and fitness coaching. Are any of these right for you? They might be; plenty of people have achieved their health and fitness goals in these ways, but that doesn't mean that you must follow rigid eating habits, unfamiliar plans, or pay to have someone coach you through the process. When it is all said and done, getting healthy has to be intuitive because at some point the focus turns to maintaining a healthy lifestyle and those plans that are overly complicated tend to cause what we call yo-yo dieting; a constant lose and gain cycle, which is detrimental to your health and your self-esteem.

This is why so many people have turned to the Weight Watchers® program over the years. The focus has always been on healthy habits that realistically fit into your life. With the added benefits of support groups, nutritional and fitness consultation, and plans designed to fit individual body types, Weight Watchers® has been a dependable means of attaining healthier lives for many people. Over the years, there have been different plans followed with this program. Currently, Weight Watchers® is using what is called SmartPoints™ to help you achieve your healthy eating goals.

How Does the Weight Watchers® Plan Work?

In the simplest of terms, the Smart Points™ plan helps you make healthy choices, and teaches you how to fit those decadent treats into your life in a way that is enjoyable without being detrimental to your body. The SmartPoints™ plan uses an algorithm that combines calorie content, saturated fats, sugars, and proteins to assign each food a point value.

When you sign up for Weight Watchers® you are taught how to calculate the number of Points™ meant to help you achieve your health goals. This will be different for each person based upon individual circumstances. From there, you choose which food you want to eat based upon a point value assigned to each food. There are no foods that are forbidden; you simply eat to satisfy your daily point limits. Foods that are nutrient rich and filling have fewer Points™ than empty calories.

How Will This Book Help Me Achieve My Goals?

You, like so many others, probably feel there isn't always time to prepare a whole meal that satisfies your dietary plan. You might end up settling for a standby, that eventually you will grow tired of, or you might reach for something that isn't as healthy as you would like it to be. These are the two paths to diet sabotage. This book is designed to help you create healthy meals that you can eat while on the Weight Watchers® plan, that are as easy on your time schedule as they are on your waistline. Each recipe can be prepared in thirty minutes or less. This means you can walk through the door and have a home cooked meal on the table in the same time it would take you to make a sandwich and open a bag of chips.

When choosing recipes for this book, we took into consideration that some meals you will want to have a lower point value, while for others you might want to "splurge" a little. Each recipe in this book is nutritious, and the point value ranges from one to ten, allowing you to plan your meals around the other aspects of your life. It doesn't get any simpler than this.

Tips and Tricks

You will notice that some of the recipes call for ingredients that are already cooked, for example cooked chicken or cooked rice. When you can, plan for one or two days a week when you precook some of you most commonly used ingredients. Make an extra-large batch of rice or throw a chicken in the slow cooker, so you can portion it out for meals through the week or next few days.

You will notice that some of the recipes appear to have more than five ingredients. This is because some things such as cooking oil or spray and basic seasonings are included in almost anything that you make, and you are likely to have these items on hand to easily add to your dishes. Also, many of the spices really are optional. If something calls for dill and you don't care for it, simply omit or substitute. The top portion of each recipe contains the five ingredients that are the bones of the recipe. The bottom portion is basic spices and oils.

Speaking of spices and herbs, fresh is best. Whenever you can, choose fresh herbs for your dishes. They add flavor and freshness that is unique from what you get with dried ones.

Keep healthy snacks on hand. Fruits and vegetables are basically limitless on the Weight Watchers® plan. You can eat them any time until you are completely satisfied, without digging too far into your point allowance.

Keep it interesting. This is a great plan for variety and you should take advantage of it. Nutritious foods abound, enjoy all of them that you can.

Quick and Easy Breakfasts

Breakfast is an important meal and usually our favorite meal as we start the day. Some people skip this meal because they have no time to prepare it. In this chapter, you'll find breakfast recipes that will help you to make quick and tasty meals within 30 minutes and less, to energize you throughout the day. The meals are healthy and mouthwatering for all weight Watchers® out there. Start your day feeling strong and it will brighten the day ahead and everything you do as you keep your weight down.

Oatmeal Muffin with Applesauce

Serves: 1
4 SmartPoints™

Ingredients:
4 teaspoons non-fat milk
3 teaspoons wheat bran
3 teaspoons whole wheat flour
2 teaspoons rolled oats (not instant)
2 teaspoons brown sugar
2 teaspoons applesauce (unsweetened)
2 teaspoons egg beaters
¼ teaspoon baking powder
¼ teaspoon cinnamon powder
Cooking spray

Directions:
1. Mix all the ingredients together until just combined. Spray a container (such as a medium-sized ramekin) with nonstick cooking spray. Pour the mixture into the container.
2. Microwave on high for 1 minute or 90 seconds. Allow it to cool, and then serve.

Nutritional Information:
Calories 100, Total Fat 0.5 g, Saturated Fat 0 g, Total Carbohydrate 20.8 g, Dietary Fiber 3.2 g, Sugars 2.0 g, , Protein 3.2 g

Weight Watchers® Pancakes

Serves: 2 (6 pancakes)
1 SmartPoints™

Ingredients:
¾ cup whole wheat flour
⅓ cup applesauce, unsweetened
½ cup buttermilk (low-fat) or skim milk
1 egg white, lightly beaten
Cooking spray (preferably butter flavored)
½ tablespoon baking powder
½ tablespoon cinnamon powder
1 ½ teaspoons non-calorie artificial sweetener
½ teaspoon lemon juice

Directions:
1. Start by mixing all the ingredients together until smooth. (If you are using skim milk instead of buttermilk, you can mix the lemon juice with the milk and let it stand for 5 minutes before adding it to the batter.)
2. Check whether the batter is too thick for you. If that is the case, keep adding 1 tablespoon of water as you mix until you get the desired consistency.
3. Spray a large, non-stick skillet with cooking spray, preferably butter flavored.
4. Take two heaping tablespoons of the batter and pour them into the non-stick skillet. Spread out each pancake slightly, and cook them just the way you would any other pancakes.
5. Flip the pancakes to cook on the other side. Serve.

Nutritional Information:

Calories 185, Total Fat 1.2 g, Saturated Fat 0.3 g, Total Carbohydrates 39.5 g, Dietary Fiber 6.3 g, Sugars 12.9 g, Protein 7.9 g

Egg, Bacon, and Hash Browns

Serves: 4
4 SmartPoints™

Ingredients:
4 hash brown patties, frozen
6 egg whites
2 large eggs
3 ounces Canadian bacon or turkey bacon, finely chopped
Cooking spray
1 tablespoon scallion (the green part), minced
⅛ teaspoon black pepper to taste
⅛ teaspoon table salt to taste

<u>Optional:</u>
8 teaspoons hot and spicy ketchup
⅛ teaspoon hot pepper sauce

Directions:
1. Coat a large nonstick skillet with cooking spray.
2. Place the hash brown patties on the skillet and cook over medium heat. Start with one side and cook until they become golden brown, about 7 to 9 minutes.
3. Flip the patties on the other side and cook them until they become golden brown, about 5 minutes.
4. In the meantime, coat another large nonstick skillet with cooking spray and heat it over medium-low heat.

5. Take a large bowl and beat together the 6 egg whites, 2 eggs, chopped Canadian bacon or turkey bacon, minced scallion, the hot pepper sauce (optional), salt, and pepper. Pour the mixture into the skillet and increase the heat to medium.
6. Allow the eggs to set partially and then scramble them using a spatula. When the eggs have set properly, remove the pan from the heat and cover it with a lid until the hash browns have cooked.
7. Place one hash brown patty on each of 4 serving plates. Divide the egg mixture into 4 portions. Top each hash patty with a portion of the egg mixture, and 2 teaspoons of ketchup.
8. Season with salt and pepper if you like, and then serve.

Nutritional Information:
Calories 85, Total Fat 4.0 g, Saturated Fat 1.3 g, Total Carbohydrate 0.9 g, Dietary Fiber 0.1 g, Sugars 0 g, Protein 10.6 g

Avocado and Pear Smoothie

Serves: 4
4 SmartPoints™

Ingredients:
1 Hass avocado, ripe and firm
1 cup pear juice, unsweetened
½ cup Greek yogurt (nonfat)
2 tablespoons honey
½ teaspoon vanilla extract
2 cups ice cubes

Directions:
1. Cut the avocado in half.
2. Remove the pit and use a spoon to scoop the avocado into a blender.
3. Add the pear juice, yogurt, honey, and vanilla to the blender and puree until the mixture becomes smooth. Add the ice cubes and blend again, and you have a smoothie for your breakfast.
4. Pour the smoothie into 4 glasses and serve.

Nutritional Information:
Calories 160, Total Fat 7.4 g, Saturated Fat 2.8 g, Total Carbohydrate 3.4 g, Dietary Fiber 3.4 g, Sugars 0.6 g, Protein 4.0 g

Homemade Strawberry Bruschetta

Serves: 4
5 SmartPoints™

Ingredients:
4 thick slices whole wheat bread
5 tablespoons light brown sugar
2 teaspoons lemon juice
3 cups fresh strawberries, diced
4 tablespoons cream cheese (reduced fat)

Directions:
1. Toast the 4 slices of bread in a toaster.
2. Heat a large nonstick skillet over high heat. Add the brown sugar and lemon juice. Cook, stirring regularly, until the sugar has melted. Within 30 seconds to 1 minute the mixture will start to bubble.
3. Add the fresh strawberries, stirring often until the berries are heated through and the juices come out, which should take about another 30 seconds to 1 minute. If more time is needed to get the desired results, then allow it.
4. Remove from the heat. Take each slice of toast and spread 1 tablespoon of light cream cheese on. Top with the cooked berries and enjoy.

Nutritional Information:
Calories 166, Total Fat 3.0 g, Saturated Fat 0.2 g, Total Carbohydrate 38.0 g, Dietary Fiber 4.0 g, Sugars 15.6 g, Protein 5.0 g

Gluten Free Muffins with Lemon Poppy Seeds

Serves: 12
5 SmartPoints™

Ingredients:
½ cup sugar
2 eggs
¼ cup applesauce, unsweetened
1 teaspoon vanilla extract
1 large lemon, zest and juiced
¾ cup plain Greek yogurt (fat free)
½ cup white rice flour
½ cup oat flour
⅓ cup brown rice flour
2 teaspoon baking powder
½ teaspoon baking soda
½ teaspoon salt
2 tablespoon poppy seeds
2 tablespoon almonds, sliced

Directions:
1. Preheat the oven to 350°F.
2. Either grease a muffin tin lightly, or line it with muffin papers.
3. In a large bowl, cream the following ingredients together: sugar, eggs, applesauce, and vanilla extract. Add the lemon zest to the mixture as well as the lemon juice and Greek yogurt. Mix all the ingredients until they are well combined.

4. Add the white rice flour, oat flour and brown rice flour, baking powder, baking soda, and salt. Mix until the ingredients have been well combined. Put in the poppy seeds and mix them with the other ingredients.
5. Divide the batter among the muffin cups. Sprinkle the almonds on top. Bake for about 20 minutes, or until you insert a toothpick at the center of each muffin, and it comes out clean.

Nutritional Information:

Calories 132, Total Fat 3.0 g, Saturated Fat 0.5 g, Total Carbohydrate 22.0 g, Dietary Fiber 1.0 g, Sugars 10.0 g, Protein 5.0 g

Hash Browns Omelet

Serves: 4
6 SmartPoints™

Ingredients:
6 slices bacon
2 cups hash browns, frozen, or chopped potatoes
½ cup onion, chopped
½ cup green pepper, chopped
4 eggs
¼ cup milk
1 cup cheese, grated
Salt and pepper to taste

Directions:
1. Start by cooking the bacon slices in a heavy skillet until they become crispy. Remove them from the pan and set them aside to cool.
2. Mix the hash browns or chopped potatoes, onion and green pepper in the same skillet where you cooked the bacon. The pan will have bacon drippings to cook the mixture.
3. Cook over low heat until the underside of the mixture becomes brown and crispy.
4. Blend the 4 eggs with the milk and then pour this mixture over the potato mixture. Top with the grated cheese and cooked bacon.
5. Cover the skillet with a lid and cook the mixture over low heat for about 20 minutes or until the egg is cooked. Remove from the heat.
6. Cut the omelet into wedges. Sprinkle with salt and pepper to taste. Serve.

Nutritional Information:

Calories 514, Total Fat 34.9 g, Saturated Fat 12.4 g, Total Carbohydrate 30.4 g, Dietary Fiber 2.8 g, Sugars 2.4 g, Protein 19.0 g

Raisin Bread with Pineapple

Serves: 1
4 SmartPoints™

Ingredients:
1 egg (medium)
¼ cup canned pineapple (no sugar added), crushed
¼ teaspoon cinnamon powder, divided
1 slice raisin bread

Directions:
1. Beat the egg in a shallow dish. Add half of the cinnamon and combine.
2. Drain the juice from the pineapple into the egg mixture and beat it again. Prick the slice of bread with a fork on both sides and soak the slice in the egg mixture. Turn the bread many times so it can absorb a lot of egg mixture.
3. Gently transfer the slice of bread to a nonstick baking sheet. Take the drained pineapple and the remaining cinnamon powder and spread it on the bread together with the remaining egg mixture. Bake at 400°F for about 20 minutes, and serve warm.

Nutritional Information:
Calories 168, Total Fat 5.6 g, Saturated Fat 2.1 g, Total Carbohydrate 22.1 g, Dietary Fiber 1.9 g, Sugars 12.2 g, Protein 7.6 g

Coconut and Raspberry Smoothie

Serves: 1
2 SmartPoints™

Ingredients:
1 cup vanilla coconut milk (unsweetened)
1 cup crushed ice cubes
¾ cup frozen raspberries (unsweetened)
⅛ teaspoon coconut extract
2 packets calorie-free sweetener (i.e. Truvia or Splenda)

Directions:
1. Partially thaw the frozen raspberries.
2. Place all the ingredients in a blender and mix at high speed until smooth. Serve in a glass and enjoy.

Nutritional Information:
Calories 106, Total Fat 5.0 g, Saturated Fat 0 g, Total Carbohydrate 15.5 g, Dietary Fiber 7.5 g, Sugars 4.5 g, Protein 1.0 g

Energizing Breakfast Burrito

Serves: 4
5 SmartPoints™

Ingredients:
2 teaspoons olive oil
2 scallions, chopped
1 tomato, chopped
1 green pepper (or green chili pepper or jalapeno), chopped
2 garlic cloves, minced
2 large eggs
4 egg whites
2 tablespoons cilantro, chopped
½ cup cheddar cheese (low-fat), chopped
¼ teaspoon salt
¼ teaspoon pepper
4 whole wheat tortillas
Cooking spray (non-fat)
½ cup sour cream (non-fat)
½ cup salsa

Directions:
1. Preheat the oven to 400°F.
2. Heat a skillet over medium heat and add the oil. When the oil has heated, add the chopped scallions, tomato, green pepper, and minced garlic. Sauté the mixture for 5 minutes. Add the whole eggs and the egg whites. Cook until the eggs are scrambled, about 3 to 5 minutes.
3. Remove from the heat and add the cilantro, cheese, salt, and pepper as you stir.

4. Spray a baking dish with cooking spray. Place one tortilla on a plate and spoon a quarter of the mixture on top. Roll up the tortilla and place it on the baking dish with the seams facing downwards. Repeat this method with the remaining tortillas.
5. Bake for 10 minutes and then serve with salsa and sour cream.

Nutritional Information:
Calories 298, Total Fat 9.3 g, Saturated Fat 2.4 g, Total Carbohydrate 36.6 g, Dietary Fiber 1.7 g, Sugars 5.4 g, Protein 17.4 g

Orange Smoothie

Serves: 2
4 SmartPoints™

Ingredients:
1 ¼ cups freshly squeezed orange juice
½ cup fat free milk
8 ice cubes, crushed
2 tablespoons sugar
1 teaspoon vanilla extract

Directions:
1. Combine all the ingredients including the crushed iced cubes in a blender and puree until they become smooth.
2. If the smoothie becomes too thin, add more ice cubes and puree again until you get the desired texture. Serve.

Nutritional Information:
Calories 148, Total Fat 0.0 g, Total Carbohydrate 31.0 g, Sugars 19.1 g, Dietary Fiber 0.4 g, Protein 3.5 g

Fruit, Vegetable and Herb Smoothie

Serves: 2
5 SmartPoints™

Ingredients:
1 cup cold water
3 cups fresh spinach leaves, chopped
2 cups lettuce, chopped
1 apple, cored and chopped
1 pear, cored and chopped
½ cup parsley, chopped
2 stalks celery
1 ripe banana, cut in pieces
½ cup orange juice, freshly squeezed
Juice of 1 lime, freshly squeezed juice
3 to 5 ice cubes, crushed

Instructions
1. Put the water, spinach, and lettuce into a blender. Start the blender on low speed and puree until smooth.
2. Gradually increase the speed to high, and add the apple, pear, parsley, and celery. Blend until smooth and then add the banana pieces, and the orange and lime juices, and ice. Serve in 2 glasses and enjoy.

Nutritional Information:
Calories 216, Total Fat 0.0 g, Total Carbohydrate 53.0 g, Sugars 34.2 g, Dietary Fiber 9.0 g, Protein 3.5 g

Satisfying Salads and Soups

Raspberry Chicken Salad

Serves: 4
6 SmartPoints™

Ingredients:
6 cup mixed greens (arugula, endive, spinach, etc.)
2 cups cooked chicken, shredded or cubed
¼ cup walnuts, chopped
1 cup fresh raspberries
½ cup feta cheese

Directions:
1. Thoroughly rinse the greens and combine them in a bowl. Toss to mix.
2. Add the chicken and walnuts to the bowl and toss again.
3. At this point, you can either keep all of the ingredients in the large bowl for serving or transfer the salad to individual serving plates.
4. Top the salad with fresh raspberries and crumbled feta cheese.
5. Serve immediately while the greens are still crisp.

Nutritional Information:
Calories 197, Total Fat 10.7 g, Saturated Fat 3.7 g, Total Carbohydrate 5.4 g, Dietary Fiber 4.1 g, Sugars 0.9 g, Protein 17.7 g

Simple Taco Salad

Serves: 4
7 SmartPoints™

Ingredients:
½ pound ground beef
½ teaspoon salt
1 teaspoon black pepper
½ teaspoon garlic powder
1 teaspoon cumin
½ cup fresh corn kernels
1 cup tomatoes, cubed
1 avocado, cubed
5 cups lettuce or salad mix, chopped
Fresh lime quarters for garnish, optional

Directions:
1. Place the ground beef in a skillet over medium heat.
2. Cook until the meat is completely browned, approximately 7-10 minutes. Drain off any excess fat. Season the meat with salt, black pepper, garlic powder, and cumin.
3. In a bowl, combine the cooked ground beef, fresh corn kernels, tomatoes, avocado and chopped lettuce. Toss gently to mix.
4. Serve the salad with fresh lime wedges for dressing the salad, if desired.

Nutritional Information:
Calories 258, Total Fat 18.9 g, Saturated Fat 5.7 g, Total Carbohydrate 11.2 g, Dietary Fiber 5.1 g, Sugars 0.8 g, Protein 13.0 g

Asparagus and Stilton Chicken Salad

Serves: 4
5 SmartPoints™

Ingredients:
1 ½ pounds fresh asparagus, trimmed
12 endive leaves, trimmed
2 cups chicken, cooked and sliced
½ teaspoon salt, optional
½ teaspoon black pepper, optional
¼ cup stilton cheese crumbles
½ lemon, zested and juiced

Directions:
1. Place the asparagus spears in a skillet and add just enough water to cover.
2. Turn the heat on to medium-high and bring the water to a boil. Cover, reduce the heat to low and simmer for approximately 5 minutes, or until the asparagus is firm tender.
3. Remove the asparagus from the pan and immediately place it in a bowl of cold water for 1 minute.
4. Remove the asparagus from the water, drain well and set aside.
5. Arrange 3 endive leaves on each plate, topped with the sliced chicken.
6. Season with salt and pepper, if desired.
7. Next, sprinkle on the stilton cheese crumbles and top with the asparagus.
8. Drizzle with lemon juice to your liking and garnish with lemon zest before serving.

Nutritional Information:

Calories 181, Total Fat 7.0 g, Saturated Fat 4.0 g, Total Carbohydrate 10.4 g, Dietary Fiber 6.8 g, Sugars 0.3 g, Protein 21.0 g

Chicken and Spinach Crescent Rings

Serves: 8
4 SmartPoints™

Ingredients:
5 ounces grilled chicken, cut in strips
1 cup baby spinach, fresh
1 (8 ounce) can crescent roll dough (reduced fat)
4 tablespoons whipped cream cheese (reduced fat),
softened
⅓ cup Mexican blend cheese (reduced fat), shredded
Spices of your choice

Directions:
1. Preheat the oven to 375°F.
2. Arrange the crescent roll dough, unrolled, on an
   ungreased baking sheet. Spread the cream
   cheese on each, and then season with your
   favorite spices.
3. Place the spinach on top of the cream cheese
   and lay on the grilled chicken strips. Sprinkle with
   the Mexican blend cheese. Make the rings by
   pulling the ends of each crescent roll up and
   wrapping it around the filling. Tuck them so they
   retain the shape.
4. Bake for 14 minutes, or until the crescent rolls
   become golden brown.

Nutritional Information:
*Calories 142, Total Fat 5.0 g, Saturated Fat 2.0 g, Total
Carbohydrate 16.0 g, Dietary Fiber 1.0 g, Sugars 1.0 g,
Protein 8.0 g*

Chicken Club Salad

Serves: 4
5 SmartPoints™

Ingredients:
8 cups mixed dark salad greens
1 pound chicken, cooked and sliced
½ cup bacon, cooked and diced
2 cups heirloom tomatoes, cut into wedges
½ cup fat free ranch dressing

Directions:
1. Place the salad greens in a bowl and add the fat free ranch dressing. Toss to coat.
2. Next, add the chicken, bacon, and tomatoes. Toss to mix.
3. Serve immediately, or cover and refrigerate for up to two hours before serving.

Nutritional Information:
Calories 215, Total Fat 4.6 g, Saturated Fat 1.3 g, Total Carbohydrate 11.0 g, Dietary Fiber 1.3 g, Sugars 5.2 g, Protein 28.1 g

Roasted Caprese Salad with Chicken

Serves: 4
6 SmartPoints™

Ingredients:
4 cups heirloom grape tomatoes, halved
1 ½ tablespoons olive oil
1 teaspoon salt, divided
1 teaspoon black pepper, divided
1 pound boneless, skinless chicken breast, cooked and sliced
1 cup fresh mozzarella bocconcini
½ cup fresh basil, torn
1 tablespoon balsamic vinegar

Directions:
1. Preheat the oven to 400°F and line a baking sheet with parchment paper or aluminum foil.
2. Wash the grape tomatoes and cut each in half.
3. Drizzle the olive oil over the tomatoes and season with half a teaspoon each of salt and black pepper. Toss to mix.
4. Spread the tomatoes out on the baking sheet and place in the oven. Cook for 10-12 minutes. Remove from the oven and allow to cool slightly.
5. Place the tomatoes in a bowl and combine them with the chicken, fresh mozzarella, and basil. Drizzle the salad with the balsamic vinegar and season with the remaining salt and black pepper. Toss gently.
6. Serve immediately, or cover and refrigerate for 30 minutes before serving.

Nutritional Information:

Calories 276, Total Fat 14.1 g, Saturated Fat 5.5 g, Total Carbohydrate 3.5 g, Dietary Fiber 0.0 g, Sugars 1.5 g, Protein 30.7 g

Egg Salad

Serves: 4
5 SmartPoints™

Ingredients:
4 large eggs
2 large egg whites
2 tablespoon mayonnaise (reduced-calorie)
1 teaspoon fresh dill, shopped
2 tablespoon fresh chives, chopped
½ teaspoon Dijon mustard
½ teaspoon table salt or to taste
¼ teaspoon black pepper, freshly ground

Directions:
1. Place all 6 eggs in a saucepan and add water to cover.
2. Cover the saucepan with a lid and set it over high heat to boil. Boil for about 10 minutes, and drain the water. Place the eggs in ice water to cool so you'll be able to handle them. When the eggs are cool, remove and discard the shells from all the 6 eggs and the yolks of 2 eggs, keeping the egg whites.
3. Cut the 4 whole eggs and the 2 egg whites into ½-inch pieces with a knife or an egg slicer. Transfer the cut eggs to a medium bowl and add the mayonnaise, dill, chives, mustard, salt and pepper. Mix all the ingredients together until they have blended well. Serve and enjoy.

Nutritional Information:

Calories 106, Total Fat 7.3 g, Saturated Fat 1.9 g, Total Carbohydrate 1.3 g, Dietary Fiber 0.1 g, Sugars 1.0 g, Protein 8.2 g

Spinach, Pears and Blue Cheese Tossed Salad

Serves: 4
4 SmartPoints™

Ingredients:
4 tablespoons balsamic vinegar
4 teaspoons maple syrup
Salt to taste
2 tablespoons olive oil
6 cups mixed baby spinach leaves
2 medium pears, sliced
¼ cup blue cheese, chopped
1 tablespoon pine nuts (optional)

Directions:
1. Mix the vinegar, maple syrup, salt, and olive oil in a small bowl. Mix well until everything has combined properly.
2. Mix the baby spinach, lettuce, and pears in a large bowl and sprinkle the salad with the dressing. Toss to coat.
3. Spread the blue cheese and the pine nuts on top of the salad. Serve immediately.

Nutritional Information:
Calories 149, Total Fat 9.7 g, Saturated Fat 2.6 g, Total Carbohydrate 15.0 g, Dietary Fiber 3.6 g, Sugars 7.0 g, Protein 3.4 g

Chicken and Egg Soup

Serves: 4
3 SmartPoints™

Ingredients:
4 cups chicken broth (low sodium)
½ teaspoon soy sauce
½ cup boneless skinless chicken breast, cooked and chopped
½ cup frozen green baby peas
¼ cup green onion, thinly sliced
1 egg, lightly beaten

Directions:
1. Put the chicken stock and soy sauce in a saucepan and bring it to a boil. Add the cooked chicken, baby peas and sliced green onion and let it boil again.
2. Remove the pot from the heat and add the egg as you stir steadily. Allow the soup to sit for 1 minute so the egg can set.
3. Stir gently and serve in bowls.

Nutritional Information:
Calories 119, Total Fat 4.0 g, Saturated Fat 1.0 g, Total Carbohydrate 8.0 g, Dietary Fiber 2.0 g, Sugars 2.5 g, Protein 14.0 g

Sweet Potato Chili

Serves: 4
8 SmartPoints™

Ingredients:
2 teaspoons olive oil
1 cup red onion, diced
4 cups sweet potatoes, peeled and cut into small cubes
1 teaspoon salt
1 teaspoon coarse ground black pepper
1 tablespoon chili powder
½ teaspoon cinnamon
2 cups black beans, cooked or canned
4 cups vegetable stock
2 cups fresh or jarred salsa
Fresh cilantro for garnish (optional)

Directions:
1. Place the olive oil in a large saucepan or stock pot over medium heat.
2. Add the onions and sauté for 3 minutes.
3. Add the sweet potatoes, salt, black pepper, chili powder and cinnamon. Cook, stirring frequently, for 3 minutes.
4. Next add the remaining ingredients including the black beans, vegetable stock, and salsa. Mix well.
5. Increase the heat to medium high and cook until the liquid begins to boil. Cover and reduce the heat to low. Simmer for 20 minutes, or until the sweet potatoes are tender.
6. Serve warm, garnished with fresh cilantro, if desired.

Nutritional Information:

Calories 324, Total Fat 3.7 g, Saturated Fat 0.6 g, Total Carbohydrate 71.1 g, Dietary Fiber 16.3 g, Sugars 2.5 g, Protein 15.7 g

Roasted Cauliflower and Fennel Soup

Serves: 6
6 SmartPoints™

Ingredients:
8 cups cauliflower florets (approximately one large head)
1 cup yellow onion, sliced
1 cup fennel bulb, sliced
2 tablespoons olive oil
2 teaspoons fresh rosemary, chopped
½ teaspoon nutmeg
1 teaspoon salt
1 teaspoon black pepper
6 cups vegetable stock
½ cup pancetta, diced

Directions:
1. Preheat the oven to 450°F and line a baking sheet with aluminum foil.
2. In a bowl, toss together the cauliflower, onion, and fennel. Drizzle the vegetables with olive oil and season with rosemary, nutmeg, salt, and black pepper. Toss to mix.
3. Spread the vegetables out on a baking sheet and place them in the oven. Bake for 15 minutes.
4. While the vegetables are roasting, bring the vegetable stock to a boil in a soup pot over medium high heat.
5. Place the pancetta in a small skillet over medium heat, and cook for 3-5 minutes, stirring frequently, until lightly crispy.

6. Remove the vegetables from the oven and carefully transfer to the boiling vegetable stock. Cover, reduce the heat to low and simmer for 10-14 minutes.
7. Working in batches, transfer the soup to a blender or food processor and puree before adding the soup back to the pot. Continue with the remaining soup until the desired consistency has been reached.
8. Serve warm, garnished with crispy pancetta.

Nutritional Information:
Calories 196, Total Fat 8.2 g, Saturated Fat 2.0 g, Total Carbohydrate 25.8 g, Dietary Fiber 9.4 g, Sugars 3.8 g, Protein 8.9 g

French Onion Soup

Serves: 6
5 SmartPoints™

Ingredients:
Cooking spray, preferably butter flavored
2 large sweet onions, sliced
2 large red onions, sliced
1 bay leaf
4 garlic cloves, minced
1 teaspoon fresh thyme, chopped
½ cup red wine
1 tablespoon Worcestershire sauce
1 tablespoon balsamic vinegar
1 teaspoon salt
½ teaspoon pepper, freshly ground
6 cups fat free beef broth
¼ cup fresh chives, or scallions, minced
6 slices whole wheat bread, light
1 cup cheese (preferably Fontina), shredded

Directions:
1. Spray a large saucepan with nonfat cooking spray, preferably butter flavored, and place it over medium-high heat.
2. Add the sliced sweet onions and red onions. Toss them lightly and cover. Reduce the heat to medium and cook until soft. Stir regularly until the mixture starts to brown, which should take about 6-8 minutes.
3. Add the bay leaf, garlic, and thyme, and continue cooking, uncovered. Stir regularly, about 3-4 minutes.

39

4. Pour in the red wine, Worcestershire sauce, vinegar, salt, and pepper and stir thoroughly. Increase the heat to medium-high and bring the mixture to simmer. Let it continue cooking, and stir until most of the liquid has evaporated, about 1-2 minutes.
5. Mix in the broth, stir and let it boil. Reduce the heat to simmer and cook for another 3 minutes.
6. Remove from the heat and add the minced fresh chives or scallions.
7. In the meantime, toast the 6 slices of bread and place them in bowls. Top them with the shredded cheese. Spoon the soup over the cheese and bread and serve.

Nutritional Information:
Calories 138, Total Fat 6.0 g, Total Carbohydrate 18.0 g, Dietary Fiber 4.0 g, Protein 15.0 g

Oyster Mushroom Egg Drop Soup

Serves: 4
5 SmartPoints™

Ingredients:
4 cups chicken stock
5 wonton wrappers
1 cup oyster mushrooms, thinly sliced
2 eggs, beaten
1 teaspoon soy sauce
½ teaspoon salt
1 teaspoon white pepper
Scallions, sliced for garnish (optional)
Lime slices for garnish (optional)

Directions:
1. Place the chicken stock in a soup pan and bring it to a boil over medium-high heat. Once the stock comes to a boil, reduce the heat to medium low.
2. While the stock is coming to a boil, lay the wonton wrappers out on the counter and slice them into ½-inch thick pieces.
3. Add the mushrooms and sliced wonton wrappers to the chicken stock and cook for 1-2 minutes.
4. In a bowl, combine the beaten eggs, soy sauce, salt, and white pepper. Whisk together.
5. Slowly pour the egg mixture into the soup, whisking constantly to create thin strips of cooked egg throughout the soup. Cook for an additional 1-2 minutes.
6. Remove the soup from the heat and serve warm, garnished with scallions and lime, if desired.

Nutritional Information:

Calories 151, Total Fat 5.3 g, Saturated Fat 1.6 g, Total Carbohydrate 15.1 g, Dietary Fiber 0.5 g, Sugars 3.9 g, Protein 10.4 g

Chicken

Honey Sesame Chicken

Serves: 4
6 SmartPoints™

Ingredients:
1 pound boneless, skinless chicken breast
2 teaspoons coconut oil
½ teaspoon salt
1 teaspoon coarse ground black pepper
½ teaspoon cayenne powder
1 tablespoon freshly grated ginger
2 tablespoons honey
¼ cup soy sauce
2 teaspoons sesame oil
1 tablespoon sesame seeds, toasted (optional)
Fresh lemongrass for garnish, optional
Cooked rice for serving (optional)

Directions:
1. Using a meat mallet, flatten the chicken until it is approximately ¼ inch thick.
2. Melt the coconut oil in a skillet over medium heat.
3. Season the chicken with salt, black pepper, and cayenne powder. Cook the chicken in the skillet for 4-5 minutes per side, or until it is no longer pink in the center.
4. In a small bowl, combine the fresh ginger, honey, soy sauce, and sesame oil. Mix well and pour the sauce over the chicken.

5. Continue cooking, just until the liquid begins to bubble, approximately 1-2 minutes.
6. Remove from the heat and serve warm, garnished with sesame seeds and lemongrass, if desired.

Nutritional Information:

Calories 210, Total Fat 7.5 g, Saturated Fat 3.1 g, Total Carbohydrate 8.9 g, Dietary Fiber 0.0 g, Sugars 8.7 g, Protein 25.9 g

Orange Chicken

Serves: 4
3 SmartPoints™

Ingredients:
2 teaspoons olive oil or cooking spray
¾ cup sweet yellow onion, sliced
1 cup red bell pepper, sliced
1 pound boneless, skinless chicken breast, cubed
½ teaspoon salt
1 teaspoon coarse ground black pepper
1 teaspoon garlic powder
¼ cup low sugar orange marmalade
2 tablespoons soy sauce
Cooked rice for serving (optional)

Directions:
1. Heat the olive oil or cooking spray in a skillet over medium heat.
2. Place the onion and red bell pepper in the skillet and cook for 3-5 minutes, or until the vegetables are just starting to become tender. Remove from the skillet and set aside.
3. Season the chicken with the salt, black pepper and garlic powder. Add the chicken to the skillet and cook, stirring occasionally, for 5-7 minutes.
4. While the chicken is cooking, combine the marmalade and soy sauce. Mix well and then add to the chicken. Toss to coat.

5. Add the vegetables back into the skillet and continue to cook for an additional 5-7 minutes, or until the chicken is cooked through.
6. Remove from the heat and serve warm with cooked rice, if desired.

Nutritional Information:

Calories 173, Total Fat 3.1 g, Saturated Fat 0.8 g, Total Carbohydrate 8.4 g, Dietary Fiber 0.9 g, Sugars 4.6 g, Protein 26.4 g

Cajun Chicken and Sweet Potato Hash

Serves: 4
5 SmartPoints™

Ingredients:
2 teaspoons olive oil or cooking spray
4 cups sweet potatoes, peeled and shredded
1 cup sweet yellow onion, diced
1 cup red bell pepper, diced
1 teaspoon salt
1 teaspoon black pepper
1 teaspoon Cajun seasoning mix
2 cups boneless skinless chicken breast, cooked and shredded
2 cups tomatoes, chopped
Fresh scallions, sliced for garnish (optional)

Directions:
1. Heat the olive oil or cooking spray in a large skillet over medium-high heat.
2. In a bowl, combine the sweet potatoes, onion, and red bell pepper. Toss to mix.
3. Add the vegetable mixture to the skillet and cook for 5-7 minutes, stirring frequently.
4. Season the vegetables with salt, black pepper and Cajun seasoning. Using a spatula, press the vegetables firmly into the bottom of the pan. Reduce the heat to medium and let them cook, without disturbing them, for 5-7 minutes, or until a crust begins to form on the bottom of the vegetables.

5. Add the chicken and tomatoes. Toss gently to mix and cook and additional 5-7 minutes, or until the chicken is heated through and the vegetables are tender.
6. Remove from the heat and serve warm, garnished with fresh scallions if desired.

Nutritional Information:
Calories 242, Total Fat 3.6 g, Saturated Fat 0.9 g, Total Carbohydrate 24.0 g, Dietary Fiber 3.9 g, Sugars 0.8 g, Protein 28.1 g

Fajita Casserole

Serves: 4
5 SmartPoints™

Ingredients:
½ teaspoon salt
1 teaspoon coarse ground black pepper
1 teaspoon cumin
½ teaspoon cayenne powder
½ teaspoon smoked paprika
Cooking spray
1 pound chicken breast tenders
2 cups yellow and green bell peppers, sliced
1 cup red onion, sliced
1 cup stewed tomatoes, chopped, juice included
¾ cup queso fresco cheese, crumbled
Fresh cilantro for garnish (optional)

Directions:
1. Combine the salt, black pepper, cumin, cayenne powder and smoked paprika. Set aside.
2. Preheat the oven to 375°F and spray an 8x8 or larger baking dish with cooking spray.
3. Arrange the chicken tenders in an even layer in the baking dish and season liberally with at least half of the seasoning mixture.
4. Place the bell peppers and onions over the chicken, followed by the stewed tomatoes.
5. Add any remaining seasoning mixture to the top of the peppers and onions.
6. Sprinkle the queso fresco cheese over the top and place the pan in the oven.

7. Bake uncovered for 25-30 minutes, or until the chicken is cooked through.
8. Remove from the oven and let sit for 5 minutes.
9. Serve warm, garnished with fresh cilantro, if desired.

Nutritional Information:
Calories 233, Total Fat 7.7 g, Saturated Fat 3.8 g, Total Carbohydrate 8.7 g, Dietary Fiber 2.0 g, Sugars 1.5 g, Protein 31.4 g

Baked Artichoke Chicken

Serves: 4
3 SmartPoints™

Ingredients:
1 pound chicken breast tenders
Cooking spray
1 teaspoon salt
1 teaspoon coarse ground black pepper
1 cup jarred artichoke hearts
1 cup heirloom tomatoes, chopped
3 cloves garlic, crushed and minced
½ cup fresh basil, torn
1 tablespoon olive oil

Directions:
1. Preheat the oven to 375°F and spray an 8x8 or larger baking dish.
2. Place the chicken tenders in an even layer in the baking dish and season with the salt and coarse ground black pepper.
3. Combine the artichoke hearts, tomatoes, garlic, and basil in a bowl. Drizzle in the olive oil and toss to mix.
4. Spread the artichoke mixture over the chicken.
5. Place in the oven and bake for 25-30 minutes, or until the chicken is cooked through.
6. Remove from the oven and let rest at least 5 minutes before serving.

Nutritional Information:

Calories 185, Total Fat 3.2 g, Saturated Fat 0.8 g, Total Carbohydrate 8.9 g, Dietary Fiber 2.0 g, Sugars 1.5 g, Protein 28.4 g

Garlic Thai Chicken

Serves: 4
6 SmartPoints™

Ingredients:
1 pound chicken breast tenders
Cooking spray
¼ cup garlic chili sauce
2 tablespoons honey
1 teaspoon salt
1 teaspoon black pepper
2 cups asparagus spears, chopped
1 cup onion, sliced
1 tablespoon olive oil
Cooked rice for serving (optional)

Directions:
1. Preheat the oven to 375°F and spray an 8x8 or larger baking dish with cooking spray.
2. Place the chicken in a single layer in the baking dish and season with the salt and black pepper.
3. In a bowl, combine the garlic chili sauce and honey. Mix well.
4. Pour the sauce mixture over the chicken, using a basting brush to evenly distribute over each piece.
5. Add the asparagus and onion to the baking dish and drizzle with the olive oil.
6. Place the baking dish in the oven and bake for 25-30 minutes, or until the chicken is cooked through.
7. Remove from the oven and let rest for at least 5 minutes before serving.

Nutritional Information:

Calories 242, Total Fat 6.6 g, Saturated Fat 1.3 g, Total Carbohydrate 17.1 g, Dietary Fiber 2.6 g, Sugars 10.6 g, Protein 28.2 g

Creamy Dijon Chicken

Serves: 4
3 SmartPoints™

Ingredients:
1 pound boneless, skinless chicken breasts
1 tablespoon olive oil or cooking spray
1 teaspoon salt
1 teaspoon white pepper
1 teaspoon fresh thyme
¼ cup Dijon mustard
½ cup low fat milk
2 cloves garlic, crushed and minced
4 cups fresh spinach, torn

Directions:
1. Heat the olive oil in a skillet over medium heat.
2. Using a meat mallet, pound the chicken until it reaches a thickness of approximately ¼ inch.
3. Season the chicken with salt, white pepper and fresh thyme. Add the chicken to the skillet and cook for 3-4 minutes per side.
4. Combine the Dijon mustard, milk, and garlic.
5. Add the Dijon mixture to the skillet and cook for 1-2 minutes.
6. Add the spinach and cook an additional 4-5 minutes, turning the chicken occasionally, until the chicken is cooked through and the spinach is wilted.
7. Remove from heat and serve warm with favorite accompaniment.

Nutritional Information:

Calories 170, Total Fat 3.2 g, Saturated Fat 0.8 g, Total Carbohydrate 2.6 g, Dietary Fiber 0.7 g, Sugars 1.7 g, Protein 27.6 g

Light Chicken Salad

Serves: 3
4 SmartPoints™

Ingredients:
2 pieces boneless chicken breast
2 celery stalks, finely chopped
1 chicken bouillon cube
¼ onion, chopped
3 tablespoons light mayonnaise
2 tablespoons parsley chopped

Directions:
1. Place the chicken breasts, half of the chopped celery, half the onion, and parsley in a medium saucepan. Cover the ingredients with water. Add the chicken bouillon cube, and cover with a lid.
2. Cook on medium heat for about 15 to 20 minutes, or until the chicken has cooked through. Remove the chicken from the heat and let it cool. Reserve the chicken broth.
3. Dice the chicken and place it in a bowl. Add the remaining celery, onions, and the mayonnaise. Add ⅛ cup of the chicken broth you had reserved, and mix well. Add more if the chicken looks dry. Serve on lettuce, as a lettuce wrap, or on bread.

Nutritional Information:
Calories 169, Total Fat 5.3 g, Saturated Fat 2.8 g, Total Carbohydrate 4.1 g, Dietary Fiber 1.0 g, Sugars 1.1 g, Protein 25.4 g

Grilled Chicken Salad

Serves: 4
6 SmartPoints™

Ingredients:
¼ cup mayonnaise (low-fat)
1 teaspoon curry powder
2 teaspoons water
4 ounces or 1 cup rotisserie chicken, preferably lemon herb flavor, chopped
¾ cup apple, chopped
⅓ cup celery, diced
3 tablespoons raisins
⅛ teaspoon salt

Directions:
1. In a medium-sized bowl, combine the mayonnaise, curry powder, and water. Stir with a whisk until well blended.
2. Add the chopped chicken, celery, raisins, chopped apple, and salt. Stir the ingredients so they get combined well. Cover the salad and chill in the fridge. Serve in a lettuce wrap, with bread, or on its own.

Nutritional Information:
Calories 222, Total Fat 5.4 g, Saturated Fat 2.1 g, Total Carbohydrate 26.9 g, Dietary Fiber 2.5 g, Sugars 8.1 g, Protein 23.0 g

Chili Turkey Macaroni with Jalapenos

Serves: 8
8 SmartPoints™

Ingredients:
2 teaspoon chili powder
1 teaspoon garlic powder
1 teaspoon ground coriander
1 teaspoon onion powder
1 teaspoon cumin
¼ teaspoon salt
1 tablespoon olive oil
1 pound ground turkey
3 cups beef broth
1 (10 ounce) can tomatoes with green chilies, diced
2 cups dry whole wheat elbow pasta
½ cup low fat milk
4 ounces cream cheese
1 cup cheddar cheese, shredded
½ cup pickled jalapenos, chopped

Directions:
1. In a small bowl, mix together the chili powder, garlic powder, ground coriander, onion powder, chili powder, cumin, and salt.
2. In a medium saucepan, heat the olive oil on medium-high. Add the turkey and cook until it turns color. Add the spices, mix them in, and allow the mixture to cook for a further 1 or 2 minutes. Stir in the beef broth, diced tomatoes, and dry pasta. Cover the pot and cook for about 8 to 10 minutes.

3. Before the pasta finish cooking, poor the milk in a pot and place it over low heat. When the milk is warm and steamy, mix in the cheese cream until it melts. The shredded cheese can then be added to the milk. Stir until it melts.
4. Empty the cheese sauce into the pasta blend and mix until the pasta is equally covered. Blend in the pickled jalapenos. Give it a taste and add more salt if necessary. Serve hot.

Nutritional Information:
Calories 322, Total Fat 15.0 g, Saturated Fat 4.8 g, Total Carbohydrate 20.3 g, Dietary Fiber 4.0 g, Sugars 11.2 g, Protein 20.0 g

Chicken Fried Rice

Serves: 4
4 SmartPoints™

Ingredients:
4 large egg whites
12 ounces boneless, skinless chicken breast, cut in ½ - inch pieces
½ cup carrot, diced
½ cup scallion (green and white parts), chopped
2 garlic cloves, minced
½ cup frozen green peas, thawed
2 cups cooked brown rice, hot
3 tablespoons soy sauce (low-sodium)

Directions:
1. Coat a large, nonstick skillet with cooking spray, and set it over medium-high heat.
2. Add the egg whites and stir frequently as you cook, until they are scrambled, about 3-5 minutes. Place the eggs on a plate and set them aside.
3. Remove the pan from the heat and coat it again with cooking spray and place it over medium-high heat.
4. Add the chicken and carrots and sauté for about 5 minutes or until the chicken is golden brown. Check that the chicken is cooked through before adding the other ingredients.
5. When the chicken is ready, add the chopped scallions, minced garlic, peas, cooked brown rice, the egg whites, and soy sauce. Stir until the ingredients have combined well and continue cooking until all the ingredients are well heated.

6. Serve and enjoy.

Nutritional Information:

Calories 178, Total Fat 2.0 g, Saturated Fat 0.8 g, Total Carbohydrate 21.0 g, Dietary Fiber 38.0 g, Sugars 2.0 g, Protein 18.0 g

Raspberry Balsamic Chicken

Serves: 3
5 SmartPoints™

Ingredients:
3 pieces boneless skinless chicken breast
¼ cup all-purpose flour
Cooking spray
⅔ cup chicken broth (low fat)
½ cup raspberry preserve (low sugar)
1 ½ teaspoons cornstarch
1 ½ tablespoons balsamic vinegar
Salt and black pepper to taste

Directions:
1. Cut the boneless and skinless chicken breast into bite-sized pieces. (You may also pound them into thin cutlets to cook through easily.) Season the chicken with salt and black pepper to taste. Dredge the chicken pieces in the flour, and shake off any excess.
2. Heat a non-stick skillet over medium heat and coat it with spray. Cook the chicken for about 15 minutes, turning halfway through so both sides can cook well. Remove the cooked chicken from the skillet.
3. Mix the chicken broth, raspberry preserves, and cornstarch in the skillet over medium heat. Stir in the balsamic vinegar. Add chicken back to the pan. Cook for about 10 minutes, turning halfway through.

Nutritional Information:

Calories 229, Total Fat 4. 6 g, Saturated Fat 0.8 g, Total Carbohydrate 21.8 g, Dietary Fiber 0.7 g, Sugars 15.0 g, Protein 24.5 g

Chicken Salad

Serves: 4
4 SmartPoints™

Ingredients:
2 ½ cups chicken, cooked and chopped
3 stalks celery, chopped
1 cup apple, chopped
¼ cup cranberries, dried
½ cup plain Greek yogurt (nonfat)
2 tablespoons Hellman's mayonnaise, light
2 teaspoons lemon juice
Salt and pepper to taste

Optional:
2 tablespoons fresh parsley, chopped

Directions:
1. In a large bowl, mix the chicken, celery, apple, and dried cranberries. Stir the ingredients and combine them well.
2. In a small bowl, mix the yogurt, mayonnaise, and lemon juice. Add the mixture to the chicken mixture and mix well. Stir in the chopped parsley, if using. Add salt and pepper to taste.
3. Serve on whole grain crackers, rice, pita bread, or make a wrap.

Nutritional Information:
Calories 220 Total Fat 5.0 g, Saturated Fat 1.1 g, Total Carbohydrate 13.0 g, Dietary Fiber 2.0 g, Sugars 7.1 g, Protein 28.0 g

Pork, Veal and Lamb

Spiced Pork with Apples

Serves: 6
5 SmartPoints™

Ingredients:
2 (14 ounce) pork tenderloins
Olive oil cooking spray
2 teaspoon 5-spice powder, divided
2 apples, cored and sliced
1 red onion, sliced

Directions:
1. Preheat the oven to 450°F. Remove any excess fat from the pork.
2. Line the baking pan with foil. Spray the foil lightly with olive oil cooking spray. Sprinkle 1 teaspoon 5-spice powder on the pork tenderloins and then place them on the baking pan. Roast the pork for about 20 to 30 minutes, or until it is ready.
3. Meanwhile, spray a non-stick pan with cooking spray and sauté the sliced onion until tender. Add 1 teaspoon 5-spice powder and mix well. Add the apple slices and sauté again until the mixture becomes soft and the onions are cooked. Cut the pork tenderloins into ½-inch slices and top them with the apple and onion mixture. Serve.

Nutritional Information:

Calories 253, Total Fat 9.3 g, Saturated Fat 3.2 g, Total Carbohydrate 9.2 g, Dietary Fiber 1.7 g, Sugars 4.1 g, Protein 31.9 g

Balsamic Pork Tenderloin with Roasted Broccoli Rabe

Serves 4
7 SmartPoints™

Ingredients
1 pork tenderloin, about 1 pound
Salt and freshly ground black pepper
2 bunches broccoli rabe (about 1 pound), trimmed
Cooking spray
2 tablespoons olive oil, divided
2 tablespoons balsamic vinegar

Directions
1. Preheat oven to the broil setting and set oven rack to the upper-middle position. Line a baking sheet with parchment paper and lightly spray with cooking spray.
2. Trim the pork tenderloin from all visible fat and cut into 8 even slices. Season with salt and pepper on both sides.
3. Place broccoli rabe on the baking sheet. Spray lightly with cooking spray. Place in the oven under the broiler for 6-10 minutes until tender and golden brown. Turn the broccoli rabe over halfway through the cooking, about 4-5 minutes.
4. Warm 1 tablespoon of olive oil in a large heavy bottomed sauté pan like a cast iron over medium-high heat. Fry the pork for 8-10 minutes, turning halfway or until cooked your preferred doneness. Take the pan off the heat and remove the pork to

a serving plate. Cover lightly with foil to keep warm.

5. Deglaze the pan with the balsamic vinegar and remaining 1 tablespoon of olive oil. Whisk the bottom of the pan to release the browned bits of flavors into the sauce. Season to taste with salt and pepper.

6. To serve, place 2 slices of the pork tenderloin with a quarter of the broccoli rabe on a serving plate. Pour a quarter of the sauce over the meat and vegetables and serve.

Nutritional Information:
Calories 317, Total Fat 16.1 g, Saturated Fat 3.3 g, Total Carbohydrate 3.8 g, Dietary Fiber 2.8 g, Sugars 0 g, Protein 36.2 g

Easy Pork Piccata

Serves: 4
5 SmartPoints™

Ingredients:
1 pound pork medallions
1 tablespoon olive oil or cooking spray
½ teaspoon salt
1 teaspoon black pepper
2 cloves garlic, crushed and minced
2 tablespoon capers
¼ cup dry vermouth
¼ cup fresh lemon juice
1 tablespoon fresh chives for garnish (optional)

Directions:
1. Heat the olive oil or cooking spray in a skillet over medium heat.
2. Arrange the pork medallions in the skillet and season with salt and black pepper. Cook for 2-3 minutes per side, or until cooked through.
3. Remove the pork medallions from the heat and keep warm until ready to serve.
4. Add the garlic and capers to the skillet. Cook for 1 minute, stirring gently.
5. Add the vermouth and lemon juice. Continue to cook while stirring and scraping the pan for 1-2 minutes.
6. Remove the sauce from the heat and immediately pour it over the pork medallions for serving.
7. Serve garnished with fresh chives, if desired.

Nutritional Information:

Calories 252, Total Fat 9.4 g, Saturated Fat 2.4 g, Total Carbohydrate 0.2 g, Dietary Fiber 0.1 g, Sugars 0.0 g, Protein 33.4 g

Slow Cooker Spiced Pulled Pork

Serves 6
5 SmartPoints™

Ingredients

Rub

1 tablespoon paprika

1-3 teaspoons ancho chili powder according to taste

1 teaspoon salt

1 teaspoon ground cumin

1 teaspoon dry oregano

½ teaspoon black pepper

¼ teaspoon cinnamon

¼ teaspoon dry coriander

Other ingredients

2 pounds pork tenderloin, trimmed

1 onion, diced

4 garlic cloves, minced

1 cup low fat beef broth

1 tablespoon apple cider vinegar

Directions

1. Mix together all the rub ingredients in a small bowl.
2. Rub the spice mix all over the pork.
3. Place the garlic, onion, beef broth and apple cider vinegar in the slow cooker. Stir a few times to mix well.
4. Add the pork.

5. Set on LOW and cook for 4-6 hours until the pork is cooked through and shred easily with a fork.

Note: pork can be used to make tacos, sandwiches, and salads.

Nutritional Information:
Calories 190, Total Fat 4.3 g, Saturated Fat 1.2 g, Total Carbohydrate 5.4 g, Dietary Fiber 1.1 g, Sugars 0.9 g, Protein 32.8 g

Curried Pork Chops

Serves: 4
9 SmartPoints™

Ingredients:
1 pound boneless pork chops, approximately ¼ inch thick
Cooking spray
1 teaspoon salt
1 teaspoon black pepper
2 ½ cups carrots, sliced
1 cup unsweetened coconut milk
1 ½ tablespoon curry powder
1 teaspoon lime zest
Cooked rice for serving, optional

Directions:
1. Preheat the oven to 450°F and spray an 8x8 or larger baking dish with cooking spray.
2. Season the pork with salt and black pepper.
3. Place the pork and the sliced carrots in the baking dish, spreading them out into as even a layer as possible.
4. In a bowl, combine the coconut milk, curry powder, and lime zest. Mix well and pour over the pork.
5. Place the baking dish in the oven and bake for 25-30 minutes, or until the pork is cooked through and the carrots are tender.
6. Remove from the oven and let it rest for several minutes before serving.
7. Serve with cooked rice, if desired.

Nutritional Information:

Calories 367, Total Fat 20.1 g, Saturated Fat 7.5 g, Total Carbohydrate 9.9 g, Dietary Fiber 2.2 g, Sugars 3.4 g, Protein 34.9 g

Spicy Pineapple Pork

Serves: 4
8 SmartPoints™

Ingredients:
1 pound cooked pork, shredded
1 tablespoon vegetable oil or cooking spray
3 cups broccoli florets
1 teaspoon salt
1 teaspoon black pepper
2 cups medium heat tomato salsa, fresh or jarred
2 cups fresh pineapple chunks
¼ cup fresh orange juice (or other citrus juice of choice)
Fresh cilantro for serving (optional)
Cooked rice for serving (optional)

Directions:
1. Heat the vegetable oil or cooking spray in a large skillet over medium heat.
2. Add the broccoli and sauté for 5-7 minutes, or until crisp tender.
3. Add the shredded pork to the skillet and season with salt and black pepper.
4. Next, add the salsa, pineapple chunks, and orange juice. Mix well.
5. Increase the heat to medium high until the liquid comes to a low boil.
6. Reduce the heat to low, cover, and simmer for 5-7 minutes, or until heated through.
7. Remove from the heat and serve with cooked rice and cilantro, if desired.

Nutritional Information:

Calories 328, Total Fat 10.3 g, Saturated Fat 2.5 g, Total Carbohydrate 22.7 g, Dietary Fiber 5.0 g, Sugars 9.4 g, Protein 37.4 g

Breaded Veal Cutlets

Serves 4
6 SmartPoints™

Ingredients
1 pound veal cutlets, trimmed
Cooking spray
1/2 cup dry whole-wheat breadcrumbs
1/2 teaspoon paprika
1/2 teaspoon onion powder
1/2 teaspoon salt and black pepper
4 teaspoons canola oil
1 large egg white
4 teaspoons cornstarch

Directions
1. Pound the veal cutlet if needed, so they are ½ inch thick.
2. Preheat oven to 400°F. and line a rimmed baking sheet with parchment paper. Spray lightly with cooking spray.
3. Mix breadcrumbs, and spices in a shallow bowl. Add the oil and mix well.
4. Sprinkle cornstarch over the veal cutlets to evenly coat both sides.
5. Beat the egg white until it becomes frothy. Place in a shallow dish.
6. Add the veal cutlets to the egg white. Massage to coat. Add the cutlets one by one to the breadcrumbs and spices mixt. Try to coat as evenly as possible.

7. Arrange the veal cutlets on the baking sheet. Bake in the preheated oven for 15to 18 minutes, until golden and cooked through.

Nutritional Information:

Calories 219, Total Fat 7 g, Saturated Fat 2.7 g, Total Carbohydrate 11.2 g, Dietary Fiber 1.1 g, Sugars 1.7 g, Protein 24.8 g

Pecan Lemony Veal Cutlets

Serves 4
5 SmartPoints™

Ingredients

4 veal cutlets, about 1 pound of veal
1 tablespoon pecans
2 tablespoons all-purpose flour
¼ teaspoon each salt and black pepper
¼ onion powder
Cooking spray
2 teaspoons reduced fat butter spread
1 garlic clove, minced
1 small French shallot, diced finely
1/3 fat-free chicken broth
3 tablespoons lemon juice
1 teaspoon dry parsley

Directions

1. Pound the veal cutlets if needed so the thickness is ¼ inch thick.
2. In a small food processor, pulse the pecan until almost powder.
3. Mix the flour with the salt, pepper and onion powder. Add the pecan powder.
4. Dredge the veal cutlets in the flour mix on both side.
5. Warm a large heavy skillet such as a cast iron over medium-high heat. Spray lightly the skillet with cooking spray. Fry the veal cutlet for 2-3 minutes on each side, or until golden brown and cooked through. Remove the veal and set aside.

6. Melt the reduced fat butter in the same skillet over medium heat. Add the garlic and shallot and sauté for 1-2 minutes until tender and fragrant.
7. Add the chicken broth, lemon juice and vinegar. With wooden spoon, detach all the browned bits of flavor at the bottom of the pan. Increase the heat to high and bring to a quick boil. Reduce heat to low. Add the veal cutlet and parsley back in the skillet for 2-3 minutes.
8. Serve warm with the sauce.

Nutritional Information:
Calories 224, Total Fat 7.7 g, Saturated Fat 2.2 g, Total Carbohydrate 4.8 g, Dietary Fiber 0.3 g, Sugars 0.2 g, Protein 32.8 g

Lamb Skewers with Cool Mint Sauce

Serves: 4
7 SmartPoints™

Ingredients:
¼ cup soy sauce
2 tablespoons honey
1 pound boneless lamb leg cut into strips
1 cup low fat plain Greek yogurt
½ cup fresh mint leaves, chopped
Salt and freshly ground black pepper, to taste
2 teaspoons five spice powder
½ teaspoon coriander
Bamboo or metal skewers (if using bamboo, soak them
in water for 20 minutes before using)

Directions:
1. Preheat an indoor grill over medium heat.
2. Combine the soy sauce and honey together in a bowl. Whisk until blended.
3. Slide each piece of meat onto a metal or bamboo skewer, stretching the strip of lamb out so that it is not bunched together on the skewer.
4. Brush the lamb liberally with the soy sauce mixture. Let set for 10 minutes.
5. Combine the yogurt and mint leaves together Season with salt and pepper to taste. Mix well and place in the refrigerator until ready to serve.
6. Season the meat skewers with salt, black pepper, five spice powder, and coriander. Place the skewers on the grill and cook, turning at least once, for 7-10 minutes, or until the meat has reached the desired doneness.

7. Remove from the heat and serve with cool mint sauce.

Nutritional Information:

Calories 243, Total Fat 8.4 g, Saturated Fat 3.6 g, Total Carbohydrate 14.6 g, Dietary Fiber 1.1 g, Sugars 12.3 g, Protein 26.8 g

Garlic Infused Roasted Leg of Lamb

Serves 8
6 SmartPoints™

Ingredients
3 bulbs of garlic
1 tablespoon lemon zest
2 tablespoons fresh thyme, chopped
3 teaspoons olive oil, divided
Teaspoon each of salt and black pepper, or to taste
3 ½ pounds boneless leg of lamb, trimmed and tied in a roast

Directions
1. Preheat the oven to 350°F. Line a roasting pan with parchment paper or foil.
2. Mince 4 cloves of garlic from one of the bulbs. Mix in a small bowl the minced garlic, lemon zest, 2 ½ teaspoons of olive oil, thyme, and salt and pepper.
3. Rub the meat with the garlic mixture.
4. Cut the top of the garlic bulbs, about ½-inch. Brush the remaining oil on the cut surface of each the garlic bulb.
5. Put the prepared lamb roast in the roasting pan with the garlic bulbs. Insert a meat thermometer in the center of roast and set to 140°F for medium-rare. Place in the oven and roast for about 80-85 minutes, or until the lamb is done to your preferred doneness.
6. When done, remove the lamb from the oven and let rest at least 10 minutes before carving.

7. To serve, place 2 slices of lamb of approximately ¼-inch thick on serving plates. If desired, squish a little of the garlic bulbs directly over the lamb with some of the pan juices (skim the fat first).
8. Serve with your favorite steamed vegetables.

Nutritional Information:
Calories 298, Total Fat 12.1 g, Saturated Fat 4.4 g, Total Carbohydrate 0.3 g, Dietary Fiber 0.2 g, Sugars 0 g, Protein 40.6 g

Pork Chops with Salsa

Serves: 4
4 SmartPoints™

Ingredients:
4 ounces boneless pork loin chops (lean), trimmed
Cooking spray
⅓ cup salsa
2 tablespoons lime juice, freshly squeezed
¼ cup fresh cilantro or parsley, chopped

Directions:
1. Place the chops on a flat surface and press each one of them with the palm of your hand to flatten them slightly.
2. Coat a large, nonstick skillet with cooking spray. Place it over high heat until the oil becomes hot. Add the chops to the skillet and cook each side for 1 minute, or until they are colored medium-brown. Reduce the heat to medium-low.
3. Mix the salsa and the fresh lime juice together and pour the mixture over the chops. Simmer, uncovered for about 8 minutes or until the chops are cooked through.
4. Garnish the chops with chopped cilantro or parsley (if desired). Serve.

Nutritional Information:
Calories 184, Total Fat 8.0 g, Saturated Fat 12.0 g, Total Carbohydrate 2.0 g, Sugars 0.6 g, Protein 25.0 g

Beef

Slow Cooked Full of Flavor Beef Chili

Serves 8
8 SmartPoints™

Ingredients
Cooking spray
1 onion, diced
1 pound extra-lean ground beef
¾ cup diced celery
¾ cup diced green bell pepper
2 garlic cloves, minced
1 teaspoon red chili flakes
2 tablespoons chili powder
2 teaspoons ground cumin
1 teaspoon dry oregano
1 teaspoon dry basil
½ teaspoon each of salt and black pepper
2 (15-ounces) can of kidney beans
2 (10.75-ounces) cans of fire-roasted crushed tomatoes

Directions
1. Coat lightly a large skillet with cooking spray. Brown onion in a skillet over medium heat for 1-2 minutes until tender. Add beef and brown until the meat is cooked. Remove from heat and drain excess fat.
2. Place all the ingredients in the slow cooker. Set on LOW. Cover and let cook for 8 hours.

Nutritional Information:

Calories 273, Total Fat 7.6 g, Saturated Fat 2.7 g, Total Carbohydrate 33.4 g, Dietary Fiber 10.9 g, Sugars 4.9 g, Protein 18.9 g

Skillet Teriyaki Beef

Serves: 4
8 SmartPoints™

Ingredients:
¼ cup soy sauce
¼ cup local honey
1 tablespoon freshly grated ginger
1 pound lean beef steak, thinly sliced
2 teaspoons sesame oil
4 cups fresh snow peas, trimmed
1 teaspoon salt
1 teaspoon black pepper
Cooked rice for serving (optional)
Scallions, sliced for garnish (optional)

Directions:
1. Combine the soy sauce, honey and ginger in a bowl. Whisk together until blended.
2. Place the sliced beef in a bowl and pour the marinade over the meat. Let it set for 15 minutes.
3. Heat the sesame oil in a large skillet over medium.
4. Add the snow peas and sauté for 2-3 minutes.
5. Add the sliced beef, along with the remaining marinade, and season with salt and black pepper.
6. Cook for approximately 7-10 minutes, or until the meat has reached the desired doneness.
7. Remove from the heat and serve immediately with cooked rice, if desired.
8. Garnish with sliced scallions (optional).

Nutritional Information:

Calories 275, Total Fat 10.9 g, Saturated Fat 4.0 g, Total Carbohydrate 18.9 g, Dietary Fiber 2.1 g, Sugars 12.1 g, Protein 25.8 g

Grilled Steak and Sweet Potatoes Skewers with Cilantro Sauce

Serves 4
9 SmartPoints™

Ingredients:
3 cups sweet potatoes, cubed
½ teaspoon chili powder
2 tablespoons rice vinegar
¾ cup fresh cilantro, chopped
¼ cup low fat sour cream
2 cloves garlic, crushed and minced
1 teaspoon cumin
1 teaspoon lime juice
1 pound beef steak, cut into cubes
2 cups red bell pepper, chopped into large pieces
1 large onion, chopped into large pieces
1 tablespoon olive oil, divided
1 teaspoon ground black pepper
½ teaspoon oregano

Directions
1. Prepare a stovetop grill and preheat the oven to 425°F.
2. On a baking sheet lined with parchment paper, toss together the sweet potatoes, chili powder and enough of the olive oil to lightly coat. Place the baking sheet in the oven and bake while preparing the rest of the ingredients, until the potatoes are firm tender. Remove from the oven and let cool slightly before handling.

3. In a small bowl, combine the rice vinegar, cilantro, sour cream, garlic, cumin, and lime juice. Mix well and set aside.
4. Using wooden or metal skewers, place the steak, sweet potatoes, red bell pepper and onion onto each skewer in an alternating pattern until all ingredients are used.
5. Brush lightly with the remaining vegetable oil, and sprinkle black pepper and oregano.
6. Place the skewers onto the stove top grill and cook, turning once, until steak reaches desired doneness, approximately 5-8 minutes per side.
7. Remove from heat and serve with cilantro sauce.

Nutritional Information:
Calories 319, Total Fat 10.9 g, Saturated Fat 4.6 g, Total Carbohydrate 30.5 g, Dietary Fiber 4.5 g, Sugars 1.6 g, Protein 25.9 g

Eastern Island Beef Stew

Serves 4
7 SmartPoints™

Ingredients:

1 ½ pounds lean beef stew cut into cubes
1 ½ tablespoons flour
1 tablespoon black peppercorns
1 teaspoon five spice powder
4 cloves garlic, crushed and minced
1 tablespoon fresh lemongrass, chopped
2 tablespoons rice vinegar
½ tablespoon low sodium soy sauce
1 tablespoon honey
2 tablespoons olive oil
1 cup red onion, chopped
2 cups carrots, chopped
½ cup poblano pepper, diced
1 tablespoon jalapeno pepper
4 cups tomatoes, chopped
2 tablespoons tomato paste
2 cups acorn squash, cubed
3 cups low sodium beef broth
1 cinnamon stick
2 cardamom pods
2 star anise pods

Directions:

1. In a bowl, combine the flour, peppercorns, and five spice powder. Toss the stew meat in the flour mixture, coating generously.
2. Mix in the garlic, lemongrass, rice vinegar, soy sauce, and honey. Mix well and refrigerate for at least 30 minutes.
3. Preheat the oven to 325°F.
4. Add the olive oil to a Dutch oven over medium heat. Add the beef, onions, and carrots. Sauté until meat is lightly browned, approximately 3-5 minutes.
5. Add the poblano and jalapeno peppers, and cook for 1-2 minutes.
6. Add the tomatoes, tomato paste, squash, beef stock, cinnamon stick, cardamom and star anise. Continue to cook, while stirring until well blended, approximately 3-5 minutes.
7. Cover the Dutch oven and place in the oven to bake for approximately 40 minutes, or until the meat is cooked through and tender.

Nutritional Information:

Calories 231, Total Fat 7.7 g, Saturated Fat 2.7 g, Total Carbohydrate 22.8 g, Dietary Fiber 4.2 g, Sugars 6.2 g, Protein 19.6 g

Creole Crusted Ribeyes

Serves 4
5 SmartPoints™

Ingredients
4 ribeye steaks, approximately 5 ounces each
¼ cup Dijon mustard
½ teaspoon cayenne sauce
1 tablespoon shallot, chopped
1 tablespoon vegetable oil
½ teaspoon black pepper
½ teaspoon allspice
2 cloves garlic, crushed and minced
2 cups green bell peppers, sliced
1 cup cremini mushrooms, sliced

Directions
1. Preheat oven to 400°F
2. In a bowl, combine the Dijon mustard, cayenne sauce, and shallots. Mix well and set aside.
3. Add the vegetable oil to a large ovenproof skillet over medium high heat.
4. Coat the steaks with the black pepper, allspice, and garlic. Place them in the skillet and sear on both sides, just until browned, approximately 2-3 minutes per side.
5. Remove from the pan and keep warm.
6. Add the bell peppers and mushrooms to the skillet and sauté for 2-3 minutes. Remove from heat.
7. Place the steaks on top of the peppers and mushrooms. Spread the mustard mixture onto each steak, and press some bread crumbs on top.

8. Place in the oven and bake until steak has reached desired doneness, approximately 15 minutes.

Nutritional Information:
Calories 205, Total Fat 8.5 g, Saturated Fat 3.6 g, Total Carbohydrate 5.5 g, Dietary Fiber 1.2 g, Sugars 1.8 g, Protein 24.2 g

Beef Medallions with Rosemary Mushroom Sauce

Serves: 4
5 SmartPoints™

Ingredients:
1 pound beef medallions
1 teaspoon salt
1 teaspoon coarse ground black pepper
1 tablespoon olive oil or cooking spray
2 cups assorted mushrooms, sliced
3 cloves garlic, crushed and minced
¼ cup dry red wine
1 tablespoon fresh rosemary, chopped

Directions:
1. Preheat the broiler and line a baking sheet with aluminum foil.
2. Arrange the medallions on the baking sheet and season with salt and black pepper.
3. Place the medallions under the broiler for 5-7 minutes, turning once, until the desired doneness is reached.
4. Remove from heat and set aside.
5. In the meantime, heat the olive oil or cooking spray in a skillet over medium heat.
6. Add the mushrooms and garlic. Sauté for 3-4 minutes.
7. Add the red wine to the skillet and cook, scraping the pan, for 1-2 minutes.
8. Remove the sauce from the heat and immediately pour it over the beef medallions before serving.

Nutritional Information:

Calories 195, Total Fat 8.6 g, Saturated Fat 3.7 g, Total Carbohydrate 1.5 g, Dietary Fiber 0.4 g, Sugars 0.7 g, Protein 24.1 g

Italian Steak Rolls

Serves: 4
5 SmartPoints™

Ingredients:
1 pound flank steak, thinly sliced in sheets
¼ cup low fat Italian salad dressing
1 cup red bell pepper, sliced
½ pound asparagus spears, trimmed
1 cup onion, sliced
Cooking spray
1 teaspoon salt
1 teaspoon black pepper
Kitchen twine

Directions:
1. Place the steaks in a bowl and cover them with the Italian salad dressing. Toss to coat. Set aside for 15 minutes.
2. Preheat the oven to 350°F and line a baking sheet with aluminum foil.
3. Remove the meat from the marinade and lay the slices out on a flat surface. Season with salt and black pepper as desired.
4. Place the red bell pepper, asparagus and onion pieces on the center of each piece of meat in equal amounts.
5. Roll up each piece of meat around the vegetables and secure with kitchen twine.
6. Heat the cooking spray in a skillet over medium high.
7. Add the steak rolls to the skillet and sear on all sides.

8. Transfer the steak rolls to the baking sheet. Place it in the oven and bake for 15-20 minutes, or until the meat is cooked through and the vegetables are crisp tender.
9. Remove from the oven and let rest 5 minutes before serving.

Nutritional Information:
Calories 211, Total Fat 8.6 g, Saturated Fat 3.7 g, Total Carbohydrate 7.9 g, Dietary Fiber 1.9 g, Sugars 1.8 g, Protein 24.6 g

Beef Soba Bowls

Serves: 4
8 SmartPoints™

Ingredients:
1 pound flank or skirt steak, thinly sliced
Cooking spray
1 teaspoon salt
1 teaspoon black pepper
1 teaspoon ground ginger
4 cups fresh snow peas, washed and trimmed
¼ cup soy sauce
1 cup beef stock
½ pound soba noodles, cooked
Fresh cilantro for garnish (optional)
Lime wedges for garnish (optional)

Directions:
1. Spray a large skillet with vegetable oil and heat over medium.
2. Add the steak slices and season with salt, black pepper, and ground ginger. Cook, stirring occasionally, for 5-7 minutes, or until the meat has reached the desired doneness.
3. Remove the steak from the pan and keep it warm.
4. Add the snow peas to the pan and sauté for 2-3 minutes.
5. Combine the beef stock and soy sauce and add them to the skillet. Cook for 2-3 minutes, or until the liquid comes to a low boil.
6. Add the cooked soba noodles and toss. Cook an additional 1-2 minutes, or until warmed through.

7. Transfer the noodles, broth, and snow peas to a serving bowl and top with slices of steak.
8. Garnish with fresh cilantro and lime wedges before serving, if desired.

Nutritional Information:
Calories 328, Total Fat 8.8 g, Saturated Fat 3.7 g, Total Carbohydrate 31.1 g, Dietary Fiber 2.1 g, Sugars 3.5 g, Protein 32.7 g

Beef Rope Vieja

Serves 6
5 SmartPoints™

Ingredients
Cooking spray
2 pounds flank steak, trimmed
2 bell peppers, trimmed and cut into bite sized pieces
1 onion, sliced thinly
4 garlic cloves, minced
1-2 bay leaves
1 teaspoon cumin
1 teaspoon oregano
¼ teaspoon salt
¼ teaspoon black pepper
¾ cup non-fat beef broth
3 tablespoons tomato paste

Directions

1. Lightly spray the slow cooker with cooking spray.
2. Add the beef, peppers, onion, garlic and spices to the slow cooker.
3. Mix the beef broth and the tomato paste in a bowl. Add it to the slow cooker.
4. Set on LOW and slow cook for 8 hours.

Nutritional Information:
Calories 262, Total Fat 10 g, Saturated Fat 3.7 g, Total Carbohydrate 7.2 g, Dietary Fiber 1.1 g, Sugars 2.7 g, Protein 35.8 g

Cool and Tangy Beef Cups

Serves: 4
6 SmartPoints™

Ingredients:
1 pound roast beef, cooked and shredded
1 cup carrot, shredded
½ cup scallions, sliced
2 tablespoons rice vinegar
½ teaspoon salt
1 teaspoon black pepper
1 teaspoon crushed red pepper flakes
8 large Bibb lettuce leaves
Fresh mint, chopped for garnish (optional)

Directions:
1. Combine the roast beef, carrots, and scallions in a bowl. Toss to mix.
2. Season the beef with rice vinegar, salt, black pepper, and crushed red pepper flakes. Mix well.
3. Spoon the beef mixture into the center of each leaf.
4. Garnish with fresh mint before serving.

Nutritional Information:
Calories 201, Total Fat 8.5 g, Saturated Fat 3.6 g, Total Carbohydrate 6.2 g, Dietary Fiber 1.2 g, Sugars 4.1 g, Protein 23.6 g

Steak with Leek Pan Sauce

Serves: 4
7 SmartPoints™

Ingredients:
4 lean beef steaks, approximately 4-5 ounces each
Cooking spray
1 teaspoon salt
1 teaspoon coarse ground black pepper
½ teaspoon onion powder
½ teaspoon oregano
1 cup leeks, sliced
½ cup dry red wine
1 cup beef stock
¼ cup gorgonzola cheese crumbles

Directions:
1. Heat the cooking spray in a deep skillet over medium-high heat.
2. Season the steaks with salt, black pepper, onion powder and oregano. Place the steaks in the skillet and sear on all sides, then remove and keep warm.
3. Add the leeks to the skillet and sauté for 2-3 minutes.
4. Next, add the red wine and reduce for 2-3 minutes, scraping the bottom of the pan to remove any steak bits.
5. Add the beef stock and return the steaks to the skillet.
6. Bring to a low boil before reducing the heat to medium low and cooking for 7-10 minutes, or until the steaks have reached desired doneness.

7. Remove the skillet from the heat and transfer the steaks to serving plates. Spoon the pan sauce and leeks over the steaks and then garnish with crumbled gorgonzola.
8. Let the steaks rest for 5 minutes before slicing.

Nutritional Information:
Calories 250, Total Fat 10.8 g, Saturated Fat 5.2 g, Total Carbohydrate 5.1 g, Dietary Fiber 0.5 g, Sugars 1.4 g, Protein 26.3 g

Fish and Seafood

Ponzu Pockets

Serves: 4
2 SmartPoints™

Ingredients:
4 cups fresh spinach, torn
1 cup zucchini, cut into matchsticks
4 flounder fillets, approximately 4-5 ounces each
½ teaspoon salt
1 teaspoon black pepper
½ teaspoon ground ginger
1 tablespoon ponzu sauce
1 teaspoon sesame oil

Directions:
1. Preheat the oven to 450°F.
2. Lay out four pieces of aluminum foil, each measuring approximately 12 inches.
3. Place equal amounts of spinach and zucchini into the center of each piece of foil.
4. Place a flounder fillet over the vegetables and season the fish with salt, black pepper and ground ginger.
5. Drizzle each portion with ponzu sauce and sesame oil.
6. Close each piece of foil over the fish in an envelope style fold.
7. Place the packets in a baking dish and in the oven.
8. Bake for 15 minutes.

9. Remove from the oven and open carefully to allow the steam to escape before serving.

Nutritional Information:

Calories 114, Total Fat 2.3 g, Saturated Fat 0.2 g, Total Carbohydrate 2.9 g, Dietary Fiber 1.3 g, Sugars 0.9 g, Protein 21.1 g

Lemon Dijon Whitefish

Serves: 4
1 SmartPoints™

Ingredients:
1 pound whitefish fillets
Cooking spray
2 tablespoons Dijon mustard
1 teaspoon prepared horseradish
1 tablespoon fresh lemon juice
1 teaspoon salt
1 teaspoon black pepper
1 lemon, sliced

Directions:
1. Preheat the oven to 450°F and spray a 9x9 or larger baking dish with cooking spray.
2. In a bowl, combine the Dijon mustard, horseradish, and lemon juice.
3. Brush each whitefish fillet with the Dijon mixture, season with salt and pepper as desired, and then place it in the baking dish.
4. Place the lemon slices over the top of the fish.
5. Place the fish in the oven and bake for 15 minutes, or until the fish is cooked through and flakey.

Nutritional Information:
Calories 99, Total Fat 1.0 g, Saturated Fat 0.0 g, Total Carbohydrate 0.4 g, Dietary Fiber 0.1 g, Sugars 0.3 g, Protein 20.0 g

Easy Glazed Salmon

Serves: 4
3 SmartPoints™

Ingredients:
1 pound salmon steaks
Cooking spray
2 tablespoons soy sauce
1 tablespoon rice vinegar
1 tablespoon shallots, diced
½ teaspoon salt
1 teaspoon black pepper
1 tablespoon toasted sesame seeds

Directions:
1. Spray a skillet with the cooking spray and heat it over medium high.
2. In a bowl, combine the soy sauce, rice vinegar and shallots. Whisk until blended.
3. Season the salmon with salt and black pepper and then brush each steak with the glaze.
4. Reduce the heat of the skillet to medium and place the salmon in the pan, skin side down (if the skin is still attached).
5. Cook for 5-7 minutes per side, or until the salmon is cooked through.
6. Remove from the skillet and sprinkle with toasted sesame seeds before serving.

Nutritional Information:
Calories 186, Total Fat 6.1 g, Saturated Fat 1.0 g, Total Carbohydrate 1.1 g, Dietary Fiber 0.3 g, Sugars 0.1 g, Protein 29.9 g

Creamy Cucumber Salmon

Serves: 4
3 SmartPoints™

Ingredients:
1 pound salmon steaks
½ cup plain low fat Greek yogurt
½ cup cucumber, peeled and finely diced
1 tablespoon fresh dill, chopped
½ teaspoon salt
1 teaspoon black pepper
1 tablespoon olive oil or cooking spray
½ teaspoon ground coriander
1 teaspoon fresh lemon juice

Directions:
1. Prepare a stovetop grill over medium heat.
2. In a bowl combine the low fat Greek yogurt, cucumber, dill and a pinch of the salt and black pepper. Mix well and place in the refrigerator until ready to serve.
3. Brush the salmon steaks with olive oil or spray a light coat of cooking spray. Season the salmon with the remaining salt, black pepper, coriander, and lemon juice.
4. Place the salmon steaks on the grill, and cook 12-15 minutes, depending on thickness, turning once about halfway through, until the salmon is flakey in the center.
5. Remove from the heat and serve with a dollop of cucumber sauce.

Nutritional Information:

Calories 186, Total Fat 5.0 g, Saturated Fat 0.8 g, Total Carbohydrate 2.9 g, Dietary Fiber 0.6 g, Sugars 2.0 g, Protein 30.6 g

Salmon Glazed with Honey

Serves: 4
4 SmartPoints™

Ingredients:
4 pieces salmon fillet
3 tablespoons rice wine (sweet)
1 tablespoon honey
1 tablespoon rice vinegar, seasoned
1 tablespoon soy sauce
1 teaspoon ginger, minced
¼ cup scallions, thinly sliced
Salt and pepper to taste
Cooking spray

Directions:
1. In a small saucepan, mix the sweet wine, honey, vinegar, soy sauce, and ginger. Bring them to a boil over medium-high heat to make the sauce. Cook the sauce while stirring regularly for about 5 minutes, until it has thickened and the flavors have blended well. Remove it from the heat and then cover it with a lid to keep it warm.
2. In the meantime, sprinkle the salmon with salt and pepper and spray a large nonstick skillet with the vegetable oil spray. Set it over high heat. Add the salmon fillet pieces and cook for about 4 minutes on each side, or until the fish is browned. Turn the fillet once halfway through. Use a spoon to spread the sauce over the fish and sprinkle with the scallions. Serve hot.

Nutritional Information:

Calories 180, Total Fat 5.0 g, Saturated Fat 0.9 g, Total Carbohydrate 5.9 g, Dietary Fiber 0.3 g, Sugars 4.1 g, Protein 23.7 g

Angel Hair Shrimp and Tomato Pasta

Serves: 4
8 SmartPoints™

Ingredients:
8 ounces angel hair (vermicelli) pasta, cooked
½ cup onion, diced
2 cups heirloom tomatoes, chopped
1 pound shrimp, cleaned and deveined
6 cups fresh spinach, torn
1 tablespoon olive oil
1 teaspoon salt
1 teaspoon black pepper
1 teaspoon crushed red pepper flakes

Directions:
1. Pour the olive oil in a large skillet over medium heat.
2. Place the onion in the skillet and sauté for 2-3 minutes.
3. Add the tomatoes and cook for an additional 2 minutes.
4. Add the shrimp to the skillet, and cook for 5 minutes, stirring frequently. The shrimp should turn pink.
5. Place the spinach in the skillet with the other ingredients and cook until wilted, approximately 1-2 minutes.
6. Add the cooked pasta to the skillet and toss to mix. Reduce the heat to low and cook until the pasta is heated through, approximately 2-4 minutes.
7. Remove from the heat and serve immediately.

Nutritional Information:

Calories 357, Total Fat 3.5 g, Saturated Fat 0.4 g, Total Carbohydrate 50.6 g, Dietary Fiber 4.3 g, Sugars 1.2 g, Protein 32.3 g

Pasta and Tuna Salad

Serves: 6
5 SmartPoints™

Ingredients:
6 ounces pasta
1 (12 ounce) can tuna, drained
¼ cup celery, diced
½ cup cherry tomatoes cut in halves
½ cup yellow bell pepper, cut into strips
¾ cup salsa, (low-salt)
½ cup mayonnaise (low-fat)
½ teaspoon red pepper, ground
2 tablespoons scallions, sliced

Directions:
1. Start by cooking the pasta according to the package instructions, but omit the fat and salt.
2. Drain the pasta and rinse it with cold water.
3. In a large bowl, mix together the pasta, tuna, celery, cherry tomatoes, and sliced bell pepper until everything has combined well.
4. In a small bowl, mix together the salsa, mayonnaise, and ground red pepper until they have combined well. Add the dressing to the pasta mixture and toss. Cover and chill. Sprinkle the mixture with scallions and serve.

Nutritional Information:
Calories 194, Total Fat 2.0 g, Saturated Fat 1.0 g, Total Carbohydrate 25.0 g, Dietary Fiber 2.0 g, Sugars 2.0 g, Protein 18.0 g

Salmon in Ginger and Soy

Serves: 6
5 SmartPoints™

Ingredients:
6 fillets fresh salmon, skinned
⅓ cup soy sauce
¼ cup brown sugar
2 garlic cloves, minced
2 teaspoon fresh ginger, minced

Directions:
1. Prepare the marinade in advance by combining soy sauce, brown sugar, ginger, and garlic together in a small bowl. Place the salmon fillets in a large resealable bag and pour in the marinade. Turn the bag to coat the salmon, and refrigerate.
2. Turn the fish from time to time so the marinade can cover it all. In the meantime, preheat the oven to 425°F.
3. Remove the fish from the fridge and seal it in a square of aluminum foil. Place it on a baking sheet and put it in the oven.
4. Cook for 15 minutes, or until the salmon is properly cooked. You'll know it has cooked through when it flakes easily when pressed with a fork. Serve immediately and enjoy.

Nutritional Information:
Calories 192.0, Total Fat 7.0 g, Saturated Fat 1.5 g, Total Carbohydrate 7.0 g, Dietary Fiber 0.0 g, Sugars 3.8 g, Protein 23.0 g

Grilled Shrimp and Watermelon Salad

Serves: 4
7 SmartPoints™

Ingredients:

For the shrimp:
10 ounces large shrimp, shelled and deveined
1 garlic clove, crushed to a paste
Salt to taste (seasoned)

For dressing:
1 tablespoon shallots, chopped
1 teaspoon water
2 ½ tablespoons golden balsamic vinegar
⅛ teaspoon kosher salt
Pinch of black pepper
2 tablespoons extra-virgin olive oil

For salad:
8 cups romaine, chopped
4 cups watermelon, diced
4 ounces soft goat cheese

Directions:

1. Take a small bowl and mix shallots, water, vinegar, salt, and pepper. Add olive oil little by little stirring until it has combined well. Season the shrimp with seasoned salt, and then add the garlic, mixing it in. You may thread the shrimp onto pre-soaked skewers.

2. Light the grill (or use an indoor grill pan if you are not using skewers) on medium to medium-high heat. Grill each side of the shrimp for about 1 or 2 minutes. Set them aside when ready.
3. In a large bowl, toss the romaine with the dressing. Divide it on 4 plates. Top with watermelon, goat cheese, and the shrimp. Enjoy.

Nutritional Information:
Calories 293, Total Fat 18.0 g, Saturated Fat 8,8 g Total Carbohydrate 12.0 g, Dietary Fiber 2.0 g, Sugars 7.0 g, Protein 22.0 g

Shrimp with Pasta

Serves: 1
7 SmartPoints™

Ingredients:
¼ cup chopped onions
2 garlic cloves, chopped
1 teaspoon olive oil
2 tablespoons white wine
½ cup cooked shrimp
Fresh parsley, to taste
1 cup whole wheat pasta, cooked
1 tablespoon Parmesan cheese, grated
Black pepper, coarsely ground

Directions:
1. Sauté the onions and garlic in a nonstick skillet with the olive oil.
2. Add the white wine and reduce the heat.
3. Stir in the shrimp and parsley, and cook until the shrimp is warmed through.
4. Add the cooked pasta and stir until all the pasta has been coated. Add the cheese and pepper. Serve and enjoy. You can serve with a green salad to enrich it and make the meal very satisfying.

Nutritional Information:
Calories 415, Total Fat 8.5 g, Saturated Fat 3.7 g Total Carbohydrate 46.7 g, Dietary Fiber 7.2 g, Sugars 18.0 g, Protein 35.1 g

Baked Shrimp with Spices

Serves: 4
3 SmartPoints™

Ingredients:
Olive oil cooking spray
1 tablespoon honey
2 teaspoons creole seasoning
2 teaspoons parsley, dried
1 teaspoon olive oil
2 tablespoons lemon juice, freshly squeezed
2 teaspoons soy sauce (low-sodium)
1 pound large shrimp, peeled

Directions:
1. Preheat the oven to 450°F. Coat an 11x7 baking dish with the olive oil spray.
2. In the baking dish, combine the honey, creole seasoning, dried parsley, olive oil, lemon juice, and soy sauce and stir well so that all the ingredients have combined well.
3. Add the shrimp to the mixture and toss it to coat.
4. Bake the coated shrimp for about 8 minutes, or until turns pink, but ensure you keep stirring from time to time. Remove from the oven and serve.

Nutritional Information:
Calories 111, Total Fat 2.0 g, Saturated Fat 0.4 g, Total Carbohydrate 6.0 g, Dietary Fiber 0.0 g, Sugars 5.0 g, Protein 16.0 g

Baked Curry Scallops

Serves: 4
8 SmartPoints™

Ingredients:
1 pound scallops
Cooking spray
1 cup onion, thinly sliced
1 cup red bell pepper, thinly sliced
1 teaspoon salt
1 teaspoon black pepper
1 ½ cups unsweetened coconut milk
1 tablespoon curry powder
Fresh cilantro for garnish (optional)
Cooked rice for serving (optional)

Directions:
1. Preheat the oven to 375°F, and lightly spray an 8x8 or larger baking dish.
2. Place the onion and red bell pepper in the baking dish, followed by the scallops.
3. Season the scallops with salt and black pepper.
4. Combine the coconut milk with the curry powder and pour it over the scallops.
5. Place the baking dish in the oven and bake for 15 minutes, or until the scallops are cooked through.
6. Remove it from the oven and let it rest for 3-5 minutes before serving.
7. Garnish with fresh cilantro and serve with cooked rice, if desired.

Nutritional Information:

Calories 249, Total Fat 16.9 g, Saturated Fat 10.7 g, Total Carbohydrate 10.7 g, Dietary Fiber 1.1 g, Sugars 1.9 g, Protein 25.8 g

Coastal Tuna Salad

Serves: 4
4 SmartPoints™

Ingredients:
½ pound tuna, canned or cooked and flaked
1 cup artichoke hearts, quartered
1 cup red bell pepper, chopped
1 cup cherry tomatoes, quartered
1 tablespoon lemon juice
2 tablespoons olive oil
1 teaspoon salt
1 teaspoon black pepper
½ teaspoon oregano
½ cup fresh parsley, chopped (optional)
Leaf lettuce for serving (optional)

Directions:
1. In a bowl, combine the tuna, artichoke hearts, red bell pepper, and tomatoes. Toss to mix.
2. Drizzle the salad with lemon juice and olive oil, then season with salt, black pepper, and oregano. Add the fresh parsley last, and toss gently to mix.
3. Cover and refrigerate for at least 30 minutes before serving.
4. Serve on a bed of leaf lettuce, if desired.

Nutritional Information:
Calories 163, Total Fat 7.8 g, Saturated Fat 1.1 g, Total Carbohydrate 5.0 g, Dietary Fiber 2.1 g, Sugars 0.8 g, Protein 18.0 g

Vibrant Vegetarian Options

Zucchini Soba Noodles

Serves: 4
4 SmartPoints™

Ingredients:
2 cups zucchini, julienned
½ pound soba noodles, cooked
2 teaspoons sesame oil
½ cup rice vinegar
1 tablespoon soy sauce
1 tablespoon honey
½ teaspoon salt
1 teaspoon black pepper
1 teaspoon crushed red pepper flakes
¼ cup fresh parsley, chopped (optional)

Directions:
1. Place 4 cups of water in a saucepan and bring it to a boil. Add the zucchini to the water and cook for 2 minutes.
2. Using a skimmer or colander, remove the zucchini from the water and immediately rinse with cold water to stop the cooking. Drain well.
3. Place the cooked soba noodles in a bowl and drizzle with the sesame oil. Toss to coat.
4. In a separate bowl, combine the rice vinegar, soy sauce, and honey. Whisk until well blended.
5. Add the drained zucchini to the noodles and pour the rice vinegar dressing over the top. Toss to coat.

6. Season with salt, black pepper, crushed red pepper flakes, and fresh parsley, if using. Toss gently once again.
7. Serve immediately or chill for several hours before serving as a cold salad.

Nutritional Information:
Calories 135, Total Fat 2.4 g, Saturated Fat 0.3 g, Total Carbohydrate 26.2 g, Dietary Fiber 1.3 g, Sugars 5.8 g, Protein 4.9 g

Perfect Garden Pasta

Serves: 4
5 SmartPoints™

Ingredients:
2 tablespoons olive oil or vegetable spray
1 ½ cups asparagus, cut into 1-inch pieces
1 cup fresh snow peas, trimmed
1 ½ cups Roma tomatoes, chopped
1 pound whole wheat pasta shells, cooked
¼ cup fresh basil, chopped
1 teaspoon salt
1 teaspoon black pepper
½ teaspoon garlic powder

Directions:
1. Place the olive oil or cooking spray in a large skillet over medium heat.
2. Add the asparagus and snow peas. Cook, stirring frequently, until just tender, approximately 5 minutes.
3. Add the Roma tomatoes and cook an additional 2-3 minutes, slightly breaking up the tomatoes with a wooden spoon to release their juices.
4. Add the pasta and basil to the skillet. Season with salt, black pepper, and garlic powder. Toss to mix.
5. Cook until heated through and the flavors are blended, approximately 2-3 additional minutes.
6. Remove from the heat and serve immediately.

Nutritional Information:

Calories 201, Total Fat 1.1 g, Saturated Fat 0.2 g, Total Carbohydrate 42.8 g, Dietary Fiber 8.4 g, Sugars 0.8 g, Protein 9.5 g

Chickpea and Spinach Frittata

Serves: 4
7 SmartPoints™

Ingredients:
Cooking spray
2 cloves garlic, crushed and minced
4 cups fresh spinach, torn
8 eggs
¼ cup freshly grated Parmesan cheese
1 teaspoon salt
1 teaspoon black pepper
2 teaspoons fresh rosemary, finely chopped
1 cup chickpeas, canned or cooked

Directions:
1. Preheat the oven to 400°F and line a spring form pan with parchment paper. Spray the sides of the spring form pan with cooking spray.
2. Prepare a skillet with cooking spray and heat over medium.
3. Add the garlic and sauté for 1-2 minutes before adding the spinach. Continue to cook for 2-3 minutes, or until the spinach is wilted. Remove from heat and set aside.
4. In a bowl, combine the eggs, Parmesan, salt, black pepper, and rosemary. Using a whisk, blend well until the eggs are yellow and creamy.
5. Place the chickpeas in the spring form pan, and arrange the spinach on them in a layer.
6. Pour the egg mixture into the pan and tap gently to even it out.

7. Place the pan on a baking sheet, and in the oven.
8. Bake for 20-25 minutes, or until it is golden on top and the middle of the frittata is springy to the touch.

Nutritional Information:
Calories 239, Total Fat 11.5 g, Saturated Fat 4.0 g, Total Carbohydrate 15.6 g, Dietary Fiber 3.3 g, Sugars 0.5 g, Protein 18.0 g

Mediterranean Stuffed Sweet Potatoes

Serves: 4
7 SmartPoints™

Ingredients:
4 medium-sized sweet potatoes
¼ cup hummus
Cooking spray
4 cups fresh spinach
1 cup tomatoes, diced
1 teaspoon salt
1 teaspoon black pepper
½ teaspoon onion powder
1 teaspoon crushed red pepper flakes
½ cup feta cheese

Directions:
1. Wash and dry each of the sweet potatoes and pierce the skins in several places using a fork.
2. Place the sweet potatoes in the microwave and cook until completely tender on the inside, approximately 5-7 minutes, depending on the size of the potato. Remove them from the microwave and let them cool just enough to comfortably handle.
3. Slice the sweet potatoes in half and scoop out the insides. Transfer the insides to a bowl and combine with the hummus. Mix well and set aside.
4. Prepare a skillet using the cooking spray and heat it over medium.
5. Add the spinach and tomatoes. Cook for 2-3 minutes, or until the spinach is wilted.

6. Add the sweet potato mixture to the skillet, and then season it with salt, black pepper, onion powder, and crushed red pepper flakes. Mix well.
7. Transfer the sweet potato mixture back into the sweet potato shells.
8. Garnish with feta cheese immediately before serving.

Nutritional Information:
Calories 220, Total Fat 5.7 g, Saturated Fat 3.1 g, Total Carbohydrate 37.0 g, Dietary Fiber 5.7 g, Sugars 0.1 g, Protein 6.9 g

Eggplant and Couscous Ragu

Serves: 4
8 SmartPoints™

Ingredients:
1 tablespoon olive oil
4 cups eggplant, peeled and cubed
1 cup onion, chopped
4 cloves garlic, crushed and minced
4 cups stewed tomatoes, including liquid, chopped
1 teaspoon salt
1 teaspoon black pepper
4 cups couscous, cooked
¼ cup fresh basil, chopped (optional)
¼ fresh grated Parmesan (optional)

Directions:
1. Heat the olive oil in a large skillet over medium.
2. Add the eggplant and onion. Sauté for 5-7 minutes.
3. Next, add the garlic and tomatoes. Season with salt and black pepper. Cook for an additional 3-4 minutes, stirring frequently.
4. Reduce the heat and let the mixture simmer for 3 minutes.
5. Spoon the cooked couscous into serving dishes and top with the eggplant ragu.
6. Garnish with fresh basil and Parmesan, if desired, before serving.

Nutritional Information:
Calories 281, Total Fat 4.4 g, Saturated Fat 0.6 g, Total Carbohydrate 53.2 g, Dietary Fiber 6.9 g, Sugars 0.0 g, Protein 8.8 g

Vagetarian Pita Pizza

Serves: 1
5 SmartPoints™

Ingredients:
1 large pita bread, thin
¼ cup pizza sauce
¼ cup green pepper
¼ cup mushrooms
10 small black olives
½ cup mozzarella cheese
2 teaspoons Parmesan cheese
1 pinch pizza seasoning or oregano

Directions:
1. Place the pita bread on a flat surface and spread the pizza sauce on top.
2. Arrange the vegetables over the sauce, as well as the mozzarella cheese. Top this with the Parmesan cheese and the seasoning.
3. Spray the cooking spray over the cheese, but do it lightly.
4. Set oven on the broil mode. Place the pizza in the oven for about 2 minutes or until the cheese is melted and golden.
5. Remove from the oven and serve.

Nutritional Information:
Calories 341, Total Fat 5.9 g, Saturated Fat 1.4 g, Total Carbohydrate 45.3 g, Dietary Fiber 5.4 g, Sugars 4.0 g, Protein 27.2 g

Cauliflower and Black Beans

Serves: 4
5 SmartPoints™

Ingredients:
1 medium-sized cauliflower
Cooking spray (non-fat) or olive oil spray
1 cup black beans, drained and rinsed
1 medium-sized tomato, diced
1 teaspoon cumin
1 teaspoon garlic powder
Salt and pepper to taste
1 cup sharp cheddar cheese (reduced fat), shredded
4 slices lean turkey bacon, diced and cooked
4 scallions, diced
½ cup sour cream (fat free)

Directions:
1. Prepare the cauliflower into bite-sized florets and steam them in a pot, or in the microwave in a lidded bowl with an inch of water.
2. When the cauliflower is tender, coat a small, nonstick skillet with cooking spray and set it over medium high heat. Add the drained black beans, diced tomato, cumin, and garlic powder. Sauté for about 2 minutes, or until the mixture has been heated through. Remove from the heat and divide it into 4 portions.
3. Place the cooked cauliflower on 4 serving bowls and then season with salt and pepper to taste.

4. Divide the cheese into 4 parts and top each serving with a portion. Microwave 1 minute each, or wait until the cheese has melted. Remove from the microwave and top each serving with the black beans and tomato mixture.
5. Top each with 2 tablespoons of fat-free sour cream, cooked bacon, and scallions. Serve and enjoy.

Nutritional Information:
Calories 253, Total Fat 6.5 g, Saturated Fat 1.3 g, Total Carbohydrate 29.0 g, Dietary Fiber 10.0 g, Sugars 12.4 g, Protein 13.0 g

Zucchini Cashew Noodles

Serves: 4
5 SmartPoints™

Ingredients:
6 cups zucchini, spiral cut into noodles
¼ cup cashew butter
¼ cup ponzu or soy sauce
1 tablespoon chili garlic paste
1 tablespoon freshly grated ginger
1 tablespoon olive oil
½ teaspoon salt
1 teaspoon black pepper
1 teaspoon five spice powder
Fresh scallions for garnish, if desired

Directions:
1. In a bowl, combine the cashew butter, ponzu or soy sauce, chili garlic paste and freshly grated ginger. Whisk until well blended and set aside.
2. Heat the olive oil in a skillet over medium heat.
3. Add the zucchini and season with salt, black pepper, and five spice powder.
4. Cook for 5-7 minutes, stirring frequently, until the zucchini is firm tender.
5. Pour the sauce over the zucchini, toss and cook for an additional 1-2 minutes, or until heated through.
6. Serve warm, garnished with fresh scallions, if desired.

Nutritional Information:

Calories 149, Total Fat 9.4 g, Saturated Fat 1.7 g, Total Carbohydrate 13.9 g, Dietary Fiber 4.1 g, Sugars 5.7 g, Protein 4.0 g

Corn Tomato Salad

Serves: 6
3 SmartPoints™

Ingredients:

6 ears of corn, husks and silk removed
¾ cup cherry tomatoes, halved
½ cup green onions, thinly sliced
2 tablespoons extra-virgin olive oil
2 tablespoons fresh lime juice, or cider vinegar
Salt and pepper to taste

Directions:

1. Cut the corn kernels from the cobs into a large bowl. Add all the other ingredients and combine well. Cover the bowl and let it to sit for 15 minutes so the flavors can mingle. Serve.

Nutritional Information:

Calories 110, Total Fat 5.4 g, Saturated Fat 1.0 g, Total Carbohydrate 15.7 g, Dietary Fiber 2.4 g, Sugars 3.1 g, Protein 2.7 g

Side Dishes and Snacks

Sesame Asparagus

Serves: 4
2 SmartPoints™

Ingredients:
1 pound asparagus spears
2 tablespoons rice vinegar
1 teaspoon sesame oil
1 tablespoon shallots, diced
½ teaspoon salt
1 teaspoon black pepper
1 tablespoon sesame seeds

Directions:
1. Preheat the oven to 450°F and line a baking sheet with aluminum foil or parchment paper.
2. Wash, trim and cut the asparagus spears in half.
3. In a bowl, combine the rice vinegar, sesame oil, and shallots. Whisk them together, and then pour over the asparagus spears. Toss to coat.
4. Spread the asparagus out on the baking sheet and season with salt and pepper.
5. Bake for 15 minutes.
6. Remove from the oven and garnish with sesame seeds before serving.

Nutritional Information:
Calories 49, Total Fat 2.4 g, Saturated Fat 0.3 g, Total Carbohydrate 6.4 g, Dietary Fiber 1.6 g, Sugars 2.5 g, Protein 1.9 g

Herbed Green Beans

Serves 4
2 SmartPoints™

Ingredients
4 cups green beans, trimmed
1 tablespoon olive oil
2 cloves garlic, crushed and minced
½ cup fresh mint, chopped
½ cup fresh parsley, chopped
1 teaspoon lemon zest
1 teaspoon coarse ground black pepper

Directions
1. Heat the olive oil in a large sauté pan over medium heat. Add the green beans and garlic.
2. Sauté until the green beans are crisp tender, approximately 5-6 minutes.
3. Add the mint, parsley, lemon zest, and black pepper. Toss to coat.
4. Serve immediately.

Nutritional Information:
Calories 66, Total Fat 3.5 g, Saturated Fat 0.5 g, Total Carbohydrate 8.3 g, Dietary Fiber 3.8 g, Sugars 0 g, Protein 2.1 g

Spinach Muffins

Serves 18
2 SmartPoints™

Ingredients
1 tablespoon olive oil
1 cup red onion, diced
1 cup fresh spinach, torn
½ cup low sodium bacon, cooked and crumbled
2 teaspoons crushed red pepper flakes
1 ¼ cup whole wheat flour
2 teaspoons baking powder
2 eggs, beaten
1 ½ cup low fat milk
1 cup feta cheese, crumbled
½ cup fresh grated Parmesan cheese

Directions
1. Preheat oven to 325°F and lightly oil 18 muffin tins.
2. Add the olive oil to a sauté pan and heat over medium. Add the onion and sauté for 2-3 minutes. Add the spinach, bacon, and crushed red pepper. Sauté until spinach is wilted, approximately 1 minute.
3. In a bowl, combine the wheat flour and baking soda.
4. In another bowl combine the eggs, milk, feta cheese and Parmesan cheese.
5. Incorporate the dry ingredients into the wet and then fold in the spinach.
6. Spoon the mixture into muffin tins.

7. Place the muffin tins into the oven and bake for 35 minutes or until golden.
8. Let cool before serving.

Nutritional Information:
Calories 92, Total Fat 4.4 g, Saturated Fat 2.2 g, Total Carbohydrate 8.6 g, Dietary Fiber 1.2 g, Sugars 1.1 g, Protein 5.2 g

Crisp Fennel and Pear

Serves 2
3 SmartPoints™

Ingredients:

1 cup fennel, thinly sliced
2 cups pear, thinly sliced
¼ cup champagne vinegar
¼ cup fresh mint, chopped
½ teaspoon black pepper

Directions:

1. Combine the fennel and pear in a bowl.
2. In another bowl, combine the champagne vinegar, mint, and black pepper. Whisk well.
3. Pour the dressing over the salad and toss to coat.
4. Refrigerate at least 2 hours before serving.

Nutritional Information:

Calories 119, Total Fat 0.4 g, Saturated Fat 0 g, Total Carbohydrate 29.3 g, Dietary Fiber 7.3 g, Sugars 15.8 g, Protein 1.6 g

Shaved Brussels Sprouts with Walnuts

Serves 4
3 SmartPoints™

Ingredients:
4 cups Brussels sprouts, shaved
2 tablespoons olive oil
½ cup red onion, diced
1 teaspoon thyme
1 teaspoon black pepper
¼ cup walnuts, chopped
¼ cup fresh shaved Parmesan

Directions:
1. Heat the olive oil in a skillet over medium heat. Add the onions and sauté until tender, approximately 2-3 minutes.
2. Add the Brussels sprouts and cook for 5 minutes. Season with thyme and black pepper.
3. Remove from heat and stir in the walnuts.
4. Garnish with fresh Parmesan for serving.

Nutritional Information:
Calories 103, Total Fat 6.4 g, Saturated Fat 1.4 g, Total Carbohydrate 8.8 g, Dietary Fiber 3.2 g, Sugars 2.0 g, Protein 2.7 g

Creamy Carrot Slaw

Serves: 4
2 SmartPoints™

Ingredients:

2 cups carrots, shredded
1 cup celery, chopped
1 cup tart apple, diced
¼ cup low fat mayonnaise
1 tablespoon apple cider vinegar
1 teaspoon salt
1 teaspoon black pepper
Fresh scallions for garnish (optional)

Directions:

1. Combine the carrots, celery, and apple in a bowl. Toss to mix.
2. In a separate bowl, combine the low fat mayonnaise, apple cider vinegar, salt, and black pepper. Whisk until well blended.
3. Add the dressing to the salad and toss gently until mixed together.
4. Cover and refrigerate for at least 20 minutes before serving.
5. Garnish with fresh scallions, if desired.

Nutritional Information:

Calories 55, Total Fat 0.9 g, Saturated Fat 0.0 g, Total Carbohydrate 12.1 g, Dietary Fiber 2.8 g, Sugars 5.8 g, Protein 0.8 g

Decadent Mushrooms

Serves: 4
3 SmartPoints™

Ingredients:
2 cups assorted mushrooms, sliced
2 cloves garlic, crushed and minced
Cooking spray
½ cup fat free cream cheese
¼ cup crème fraiche
1 tablespoon fresh chives, chopped
1 teaspoon salt
1 teaspoon black pepper
½ teaspoon thyme

Directions:
1. Prepare a skillet with the cooking spray and heat over medium.
2. Add the mushrooms and garlic to the skillet and sauté for 3-4 minutes.
3. Add the cream cheese, crème fraiche, and fresh chives.
4. Season with salt, black pepper, and thyme. Cook, stirring frequently, to blend the cream cheese and crème fraiche, for 3 minutes.
5. Remove from heat and serve immediately.

Nutritional Information:
Calories 79, Total Fat 4.2 g, Saturated Fat 2.6 g, Total Carbohydrate 3.5 g, Dietary Fiber 0.4 g, Sugars 2.0 g, Protein 5.5 g

Lemon Walnut Quinoa

Serves: 6
5 SmartPoints™

Ingredients:
2 cups chicken stock
1 cup quinoa
¼ cup walnuts, chopped
2 teaspoons lemon zest
1 teaspoon salt
1 teaspoon black pepper
1 teaspoon tarragon
¼ cup goat cheese

Directions:
1. Pour the chicken stock in a saucepan over medium-high heat and bring it to a boil.
2. Stir in the quinoa, reduce the heat to low, cover, and simmer for 15-20 minutes or until tender.
3. Remove the quinoa from the heat and fluff it with a fork.
4. Stir in the walnuts, lemon zest, salt, black pepper, and tarragon. Mix well.
5. Transfer the quinoa to serving dishes and garnish with bits of goat cheese before serving.

Nutritional Information:
Calories 193, Total Fat 7.6 g, Saturated Fat 1.5 g, Total Carbohydrate 24.3 g, Dietary Fiber 2.3 g, Sugars 3.5 g, Protein 7.8 g

Spiced Brussels Sprouts

Serves: 4
2 SmartPoints™

Ingredients:
4 cups Brussels sprouts, halved
1 cup onion, sliced
1 tablespoon olive oil
1 teaspoon cinnamon
½ teaspoon cayenne powder
1 teaspoon salt
1 teaspoon black pepper

Directions:
1. Preheat the oven to 450°F and line a baking sheet with aluminum foil.
2. Place the Brussels sprouts and onions in a bowl.
3. Drizzle the vegetables with olive oil and then season with the cinnamon, cayenne powder, salt and black pepper. Toss to coat.
4. Spread the vegetables out onto the baking sheet.
5. Place in the oven and roast for 20-25 minutes, tossing occasionally.
6. Remove from the oven and let cool slightly before serving.

Nutritional Information:
Calories 79, Total Fat 3.7 g, Saturated Fat 0.5 g, Total Carbohydrate 10.4 g, Dietary Fiber 3.9 g, Sugars 1.9 g, Protein 3.3 g

Desserts

Cupcake Brownies

Serves: 12
2 SmartPoints™

These cupcake brownies make a nice dessert especially when served with fresh strawberries. You may also top them with 2 tablespoons whipped topping such as Cool Whip™ to add to the flavor. This will cost an additional SmartPoint™

Ingredients:
¾ cup all-purpose flour
½ cup sugar, preferably brown
3 tablespoons cocoa, unsweetened
½ teaspoon baking soda
¼ teaspoon salt
½ cup water
¼ cup applesauce, unsweetened
1 tablespoon brown sugar, firmly packed
1 ½ teaspoons margarine, melted
½ teaspoon vanilla extract
½ teaspoon cider vinegar
Cooking spray (optional)

Directions:
1. Preheat the oven to 350°F.
2. In a large bowl, combine the flour, brown sugar, unsweetened cocoa, baking soda, and salt. Mix well.

3. In another bowl, stir together all the other ingredients. Pour the mixture over the flour mixture and stir just until the batter is smooth.
4. Coat a nonstick muffin tin with 12 cups with vegetable oil spray, or line them with paper liners. Pour the batter into the muffin cups until they're half full.
5. Bake for 18 to 20 minutes. To ensure that the cupcakes are cooked, prick them in the center with a toothpick and if it comes out clean, they are ready. Remove them from the oven and let them stand for 5 minutes before transferring them to the rack to cool. Enjoy.

Nutritional Information:
Calories 78, Total Fat 0.7 g, Saturated Fat 0.2 g, Total Carbohydrate 17.3 g, Dietary Fiber 0.7 g, Sugars 10.6 g, Protein 1.1 g

Banana Roll Ups

Serves: 1
5 SmartPoints™

Ingredients:
1 6-inch whole wheat tortilla
1 tablespoon peanut butter (reduced-fat)
1 teaspoon raspberry jam (sugar-free)
1 teaspoon dried coconut (unsweetened), shredded
½ medium-sized ripe banana, sliced

Directions:
1. Lay the whole wheat tortilla on a flat surface and spread the peanut butter and jam evenly on it. Sprinkle the dried shredded coconut on top.
2. Arrange the banana pieces on the tortilla. Roll up the tortilla to enclose the banana pieces. Wrap it in a paper towel and put in the microwave on high mode for 30 to 35 seconds.
3. Remove from microwave and unwrap from the paper towel. Enjoy.

Nutritional Information:
Calories 160, Total Fat 7.0 g, Saturated Fat 1.0 g, Total Carbohydrate 25.0 g, Dietary Fiber 3.0 g, Sugars 12.0 g, Protein 5.0 g

Fruit and Pudding Mix Dessert

Serves: 6
4 SmartPoints™

This is a nice treat which you can enjoy as dessert. It is easy to make and the taste is awesome. You may add ripe banana pieces or other fruits if you like.

Ingredients:
1 (20 ounce) can pineapple chunks
1 (15 ounce) can oranges
1 (5 ⅛ ounces) vanilla pudding mix (sugar-free and low-fat), preferably instant

Directions:
1. Drain the fruit juices into a bowl and add the dry pudding. This will help to mix the pudding so you don't have to add milk.
2. Add all the other ingredients and blend them well. Chill the dessert. Serve and enjoy.

Nutritional Information:
Calories 94, Total Fat 0.3 g, Saturated Fat 0.0 g, Total Carbohydrate 24.3 g, Dietary Fiber 2.0 g, Sugars 21.1 g, Protein 1.0 g

Banana "Ice Cream" Dessert

Serves: 2
1 SmartPoints™

Ingredients:
2 ripe bananas, peeled
2 tablespoons skim milk or fruit juice
1 teaspoon vanilla extract

Directions:
1. Cut the banana into chunks and freeze them. Put the frozen banana chunks in a blender or food processor and puree.
2. Add the vanilla extract and milk or juice to make soft banana "ice cream" dessert. Serve the same way you serve ice cream and layer with strawberries. You may add other frozen fruits of your choice such as mango or pineapple. You can also serve it with chocolate syrup.

Nutritional Information:
Calories 121, Total Fat 0.9 g, Saturated Fat.0 g
Total Carbohydrate 27.9 g, Dietary Fiber 3.1 g, Sugars
14.7 g, Protein 1.8 g

No Point Banana Strawberry "Ice Cream" Dessert

Serves: 1
0 SmartPoints™

Ingredients:
1 ripe bananas, peeled
3 fresh strawberries for serving, sliced

Directions:
1. Cut the banana into chunks and freeze them. Put the frozen banana chunks in a blender or food processor and puree.
2. Serve ice cream with sliced strawberries. You may add other fruits of your choice such as mango or pineapple.

Nutritional Information:
Calories 127.8, Total Fat 1.1 g, Saturated Fat 0 g, Total Carbohydrate 32.7 g, Dietary Fiber 4.3 g, Sugars 17.7 g, Protein 2.1 g

Frozen Fruit Dessert

Serves: 24
1 SmartPoints™

Ingredients:
1 can whole berry cranberry sauce
1 can pineapple, crushed
1 container whipped topping (fat free)
1/4 cup walnuts, chopped

Directions:
1. Mix all the ingredients together and combine well. Divide the mixture into 24 cupcake pans with liners. Freeze. Remove the frozen desserts and place them in a plastic bag and then store in the freezer. Enjoy one whenever you want something sweet and cold.

Nutritional Information:
Calories 63, Total Fat 0.8 g, Saturated Fat 0.2 g Total Carbohydrate 13.4 g, Dietary Fiber 0.6 g, Sugars 9.1g, Protein 0.1 g

Coconut and Cranberry Macaroons

Serves: 12, 2 macaroons per serving
2 SmartPoints™

Ingredients:
2 egg whites (large size)
¼ teaspoon salt
⅓ cup sugar
1 cup sweetened flaked coconut
½ cup dried cranberries
2 tablespoons all-purpose flour
½ teaspoon vanilla extract
Cooking spray

Directions:
1. Preheat the oven to 325°F, and coat 2 cooking sheets with vegetable oil spray, or line them with parchment paper.
2. In a medium bowl, combine the egg whites and salt. Use an electric mixer to beat at low speed for about 1 minute, until the egg whites foam.
3. Gradually add the sugar as you increase the mixer speed for about 5 to 7 minutes.
4. Fold in the remaining ingredients. Drop the batter using a tablespoon onto a cookie sheet. Bake for about 15 minutes or until the macaroons become light golden brown. Remove from the oven and serve.

Nutritional Information:
Calories 68., Total Fat 3.0 g, Saturated Fat 1.2 g Total Carbohydrate 10.0 g, Dietary Fiber 0.0 g, Sugars 9.0 g, Protein 1.0 g

Frozen Peanut Butter Cups

Serves: 12
2 SmartPoints™

Ingredients:
Fat free whipped topping (1 tube or approximately 8 ounces), thawed
6 tablespoons peanut butter (creamy)
4 tablespoons chocolate syrup (sugar-free), preferably Hershey's®

Directions:
1. Mix the whipped topping and peanut butter together.
2. Use a spoon to drop the mixture into 12 lined cupcake tins. Drizzle with chocolate syrup. Freeze, and enjoy.

Nutritional Information:
Calories 32, Total Fat 2.0 g, Saturated Fat 0 g Total Carbohydrate 3.0 g, Dietary Fiber 0 g, Sugars 2.0 g, Protein 1.0 g

Truffles

Yields 24, 2 truffles per serving
2 SmartPoints™

Ingredients:
1 cup powdered sugar
½ cup cocoa, unsweetened
½ cup fat-free cream cheese
½ teaspoon vanilla extract

Directions:
1. Prepare a baking sheet with parchment paper, and sprinkle it cocoa powder.
2. Mix all the ingredients with an electric mixer. Use a rounded teaspoon to drop the mixture onto the sheet.
3. Roll the mixture into balls and put in the refrigerator. Enjoy.

Nutritional Information:
Calories 36, Total Fat 0 g, Saturated Fat 0 g Total Carbohydrate 6.8 g, Dietary Fiber 0.6 g, Sugars 5.1 g, Protein 0.8 g

Pumpkin Pudding

Serves: 2
3 SmartPoints™

Ingredients:
1 ½ cups skim milk
1 (15 ounce) can pure pumpkin
½ box instant vanilla pudding (sugar free and fat free)
1 tablespoon ground allspice
1 tablespoon cinnamon
Add brown sugar to taste

Directions:
1. To make thick pumpkin , combine skim milk and pumpkin in a pan and stir. Add the instant pudding and combine.
2. Add the remaining ingredients and stir. Add more seasonings to taste if desired. Heat and stir occasionally until the soup is warm. Enjoy.

Nutritional Information:
Calories 163, Total Fat 0.9 g, Saturated Fat 0.1 g, Total Carbohydrate 30.8 g, Dietary Fiber 1.7 g, Sugars 17.2 g, Protein 9.5 g

Conclusion

The Weight Watchers® Program takes the guesswork out of losing weight and being healthy. This book is an additional tool for you to use along your path to better health and wellbeing. Each recipe is simple and delicious, requiring little from you in terms of time or ingredients. The goal of this book is to not only help you achieve your health goals, but to help you maintain those achievements for years to come. Now is always the right time to start or continue fueling your body with the healthiest and most delicious foods available. This book is simply a way to help you see how easily you can transform a basic list of ingredients into a satisfying meal. This is your lifestyle now: healthy and effortless. All you have to do is enjoy the benefits.

More books from Madison Miller

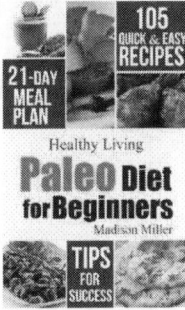

105 QUICK & EASY RECIPES
21-DAY MEAL PLAN
Healthy Living
Paleo Diet for Beginners
Madison Miller
TIPS FOR SUCCESS

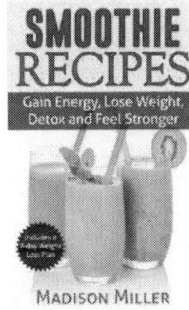

SMOOTHIE RECIPES
Gain Energy, Lose Weight, Detox and Feel Stronger
MADISON MILLER

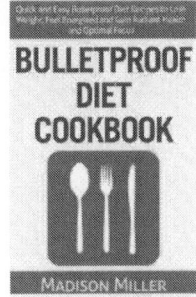

BULLETPROOF DIET COOKBOOK
MADISON MILLER

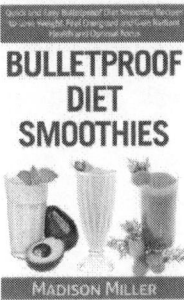

BULLETPROOF DIET SMOOTHIES
MADISON MILLER

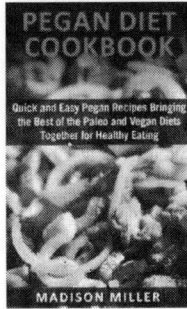

PEGAN DIET COOKBOOK
Quick and Easy Pegan Recipes Bringing the Best of the Paleo and Vegan Diets Together for Healthy Eating
MADISON MILLER

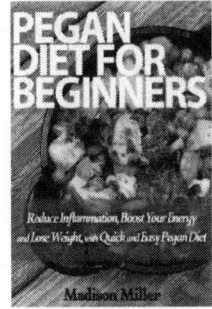

PEGAN DIET FOR BEGINNERS
Reduce Inflammation, Boost Your Energy and Lose Weight, with Quick and Easy Pegan Diet
Madison Miller

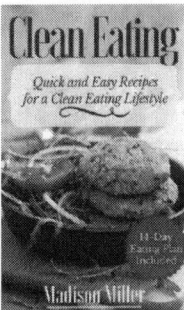

Clean Eating
Quick and Easy Recipes for a Clean Eating Lifestyle
Madison Miller

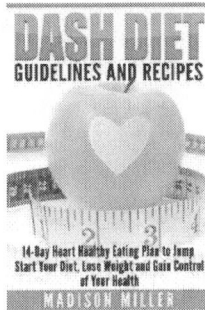

DASH DIET GUIDELINES AND RECIPES
14-Day Heart Healthy Eating Plan to Jump Start Your Diet, Lose Weight and Gain Control of Your Health
MADISON MILLER

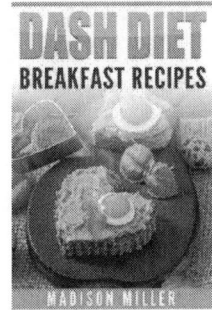

DASH DIET BREAKFAST RECIPES
MADISON MILLER

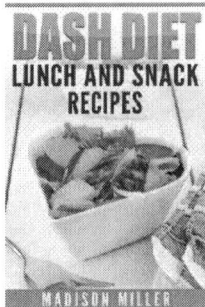

DASH DIET
LUNCH AND SNACK
RECIPES

MADISON MILLER

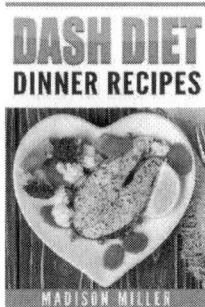

DASH DIET
DINNER RECIPES

MADISON MILLER

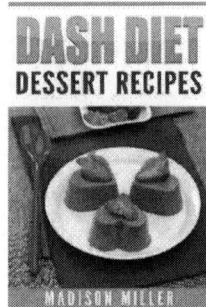

DASH DIET
DESSERT RECIPES

MADISON MILLER

Appendix

Measuring Equivalent Chart

Type	Imperial	Imperial	Metric
Weight	1 dry ounce		28g
	1 pound	16 dry ounces	0.45 kg
Volume	1 teaspoon		5 ml
	1 dessert spoon	2 teaspoons	10 ml
	1 tablespoon	3 teaspoons	15 ml
	1 Australian tablespoon	4 teaspoons	20 ml
	1 fluid ounce	2 tablespoons	30 ml
	1 cup	16 tablespoons	240 ml
	1 cup	8 fluid ounces	240 ml
	1 pint	2 cups	470 ml
	1 quart	2 pints	0.95 l
	1 gallon	4 quarts	3.8 l
Length	1 inch		2.54 cm

*   Numbers are rounded to the closest equivalent

Oven Temperature Equivalent Chart

T(°F)	T(°C)
220	100
225	110
250	120
275	140
300	150
325	160
350	180
375	190
400	200
425	220
450	230
475	250
500	260

*   T(°C) = [T(°F)-32] * 5/9

**   T(°F) = T(°C) * 9/5 + 32

*** Numbers are rounded to the closest equivalent

Printed in Great Britain
by Amazon